Manual of
diagnostic ultrasound

Edited by
P. E. S. Palmer
University of California
Davis, California, USA

World Health Organization
Geneva
1995

WHO Library Cataloguing in Publication Data

Manual of diagnostic ultrasound / edited by P. E. S. Palmer.

    1.Diagnostic imaging   2.Ultrasonography I.Palmer, P. E. S.

    ISBN 92 4 154461 9   (NLM Classification: WB 289)

TYPESET IN USA

PRINTED IN FRANCE

90/8562 - 95/10458 — Palmer/Jouve — 8000

Authors

The World Health Organization is grateful to the authors of this manual who freely contributed their time and expertise in its production:

B. Breyer
University of Zagreb, Zagreb, Croatia

C. A. Bruguera
Diagnostic Imaging Teaching Institute, Buenos Aires, Argentina

H. A. Gharbi
University of Tunis, Tunis, Tunisia

B. B. Goldberg
Thomas Jefferson University, Philadelphia, United States of America

F. E. H. Tan
College of General Practitioners, Kuala Lumpur, Malaysia

M. W. Wachira
University of Nairobi, Nairobi, Kenya

F. S. Weill
University of Besançon, Besançon, France

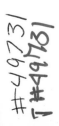
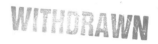

Contents

Preface

Diagnostic imaging is recognized as an important adjunct to clinical examination in the care of patients with many common illnesses. Most such imaging will be by radiography (X-rays) or ultrasound. In pursuit of the World Health Organization's goal of health for all, many of the examinations will be performed at the first referral level, where patients will be seen, referred from primary care or in need of emergency treatment. Many countries do not have sufficient radiologists or sonologists to provide skilled techniques and interpretation, and imaging may be requested, interpreted and often performed by medical officers with little or no specialist training or experience.

This manual is one of several published by the World Health Organization to provide guidance on the use of diagnostic imaging by non-specialists.[1] The use of ultrasound is increasing rapidly worldwide; it is particularly important in obstetrics, but also provides useful information about the abdomen and soft tissues. Because there is no ionizing radiation, ultrasound should be the preferred method of imaging whenever it can give useful clinical information.

The manual is a basic reference text to help with technique, recognition of the normal, and differential diagnosis. It indicates the clinical situations in which ultrasound scanning is likely to provide guidance for the care of the patient, and those in which scanning will not be reliable or helpful. The decision to scan is based on many factors and each individual patient's needs must be taken into account.

The safety of ultrasound has been a subject of considerable discussion and study. After three decades of use and the examination of thousands, probably millions, of people, the question of absolute safety is still being debated. The potential risks, if any, also need to be weighed against the benefits, particularly in obstetrics, where ultrasound provides much information that cannot be obtained in any other way.

For a small hospital or clinic, radiography (such as is provided by the WHO Radiological System) should remain the first choice of imaging technique, although ultrasound may be tempting because the equipment is less expensive and apparently less complicated. However, ultrasound cannot image the lungs, fractures or most skeletal abnormalities: its limitations must be recognized.

Ultrasound is very operator-dependent. In its report,[2] a WHO Scientific Group stated "The difficulties in making an accurate diagnosis from ultrasound images are such that the purchase of ultrasound equipment without making provision for the training of an operator is contrary to good health care practice and is unlikely to be cost effective." Proper training and experience are required, preferably with teachers who are highly skilled and who have practised ultrasound for many years. The Group concluded that a physician needs at least one month's full-time training in a busy ultrasound department to achieve even a minimum

---

[1] *Manual of darkroom technique* (1985), *Manual of radiographic interpretation for general practitioners* (1985), and *Manual of radiographic technique* (1986).

[2] *Future use of new imaging technologies in developing countries*: report of a WHO Scientific Group. Geneva, World Health Organization, 1985 (WHO Technical Report Series, No. 723).

level of expertise. This would amount to at least 200 obstetric and abdominal examinations made under supervision. For a physician to go on to become a competent sonologist, the Group recommended at least six months' full-time training in a recognized centre, and even then further experience would be advisable under supervision. They concluded that "Wherever possible, ultrasound examinations should be carried out by trained physicians", and went on to add that if non-physicians are to perform examinations, they need to have had at least one year's full-time training in ultrasound and preferably a background in radiography or nursing; they should always work under the supervision of an experienced sonologist.

The authors of this manual fully endorse these recommendations and only agreed to prepare this manual because they recognized that for many users of ultrasound there will not be experts to whom patients or scans can be sent when interpretation is difficult. This manual is not meant to take the place of proper training, nor is it meant to replace the textbooks already available. On the contrary, it is a supplement to these to help the less experienced who may not have reached the level of knowledge and skill so often taken for granted by more comprehensive texts.

The manual also provides guidance on the standards by which ultrasound equipment may be judged. There are many varieties of such equipment and too often there is no independent expert to guide the practitioner in the purchase of a unit. Particularly, there is not always information about the shortcomings and inadequacies of what may appear to be a bargain. The WHO Scientific Group mentioned above provided specifications for a general purpose ultrasound scanner (GPUS). Updated specifications are included in this manual and any product that meets them will produce quality ultrasound images. The GPUS, as its name implies, is suitable for all general purpose studies at any level of medical care and will only be bettered by much more expensive ultrasound units.

It is hoped that the use of this manual will not be limited to general practitioners, and that it will provide a starting-point for medical students, midwives and those training to be specialists in diagnostic imaging. In many places ultrasound is the only scanning technique readily available. Unfortunately, in some countries it has already gained a reputation for unreliability because it has been used by people who, as a result of insufficient training, have made many errors of diagnosis. In this way it can be dangerous. It is hoped that this manual will stimulate the interest and expand the knowledge of those who use it, so that it becomes part of their training and leads to much wider and deeper understanding of this very important imaging technique.

The authors realize that this manual will not meet the needs of everyone. Comments and suggestions will be welcome and of considerable value for a revised edition. All correspondence should be addressed to Chief, Radiation Medicine, World Health Organization, 1211 Geneva 27, Switzerland.

Acknowledgements

The authors and editor would like to record their appreciation of the unsparing help provided by Dr V. Volodin, Medical Officer, Radiation Medicine, WHO, Geneva. We were fortunate to have the thoughtful and skilled professional guidance of Dr P. A. Butler, Head, Technical Publications, WHO. Professor Asim Kurjak (Zagreb) was particularly helpful, and Dr W. E. Brant (Davis) gave much useful advice and practical help with the illustrations. The World Federation of Ultrasound in Medicine and Biology (WFUMB) gave welcome information and support. Appreciation must be also recorded for the support provided by many colleagues, in particular:

In Sacramento, Dr Gilland Dea;

In Nairobi, the staff of the Nairobi X-ray Centre;

In Philadelphia, Dr L. Needleman and Dr Ji-Bin Liu, with Mr T. L. Berry and Ms R. A. Curry;

In Rijeka, Professor Z. Fućkar;

In Tunis, Dr K. Abdesselem-Ait-Khelifa, Dr I. Bardi, Dr F. Ben Chehida, Dr A. Hammou-Jeddi and Dr R. Slim;

In Yonago, Professor K. Maeda;

In Zagreb, Mr V. Andreić.

Extra scans were provided by Professor B. J. Cremin of Cape Town, South Africa, and Dr Sam Mindel of Harare, Zimbabwe.

Without the willing assistance of all these people, it would have been difficult to produce this manual.

The staff of Illustration Services, University of California, Davis, provided many innovative ideas for the production of this manual. Particular appreciation goes to Claudia R. Graham for the illustrations and layout of the pages, and Craig F. Hillis and Rick Hayes for computer and design assistance. The scans were obtained from many parts of the world and together with the accompanying low-contrast reference images were reproduced by Illustration Services, University of California, Davis.

Glossary

Acoustic beam The beam of ultrasound waves (energy) produced by the transducer (probe). May be divergent, focused or parallel.

Acoustic enhancement The increased echogenicity (echo brightness) of tissues that lie behind a structure that causes little or no attenuation of the ultrasound waves, such as a fluid-filled cyst. The opposite to acoustic enhancement is acoustic *shadowing* (q.v.).

Acoustic impedance The resistance offered by tissues to the movement of particles caused by ultrasound waves. It is equal to the product of the density of the tissue and the speed of the ultrasound wave in the tissue. It is because tissues have different impedances that ultrasound can provide images of the part of the body being scanned.

Acoustic shadowing The decreased echogenicity of tissues that lie behind a structure that causes marked attenuation of the ultrasound waves. The opposite to acoustic shadowing is acoustic *enhancement* (q.v.).

Acoustic window A tissue or structure that offers little obstruction to the ultrasound waves, and can therefore be used as a route to obtain images of a deeper structure. For example, when the bladder is full of urine it forms an excellent acoustic window through which the pelvic structures may be imaged. Similarly, it is better to image the right kidney through the liver than through the thick muscles of the back. In this case the liver is the acoustic window.

Anechogenic (anechoic) Without echoes; echo-free. For example, normal urine and bile are anechogenic, i.e. they have no internal echoes.

Artefact A feature appearing in an ultrasound image that does not correspond to or represent an actual anatomical or pathological structure, either in shape, direction or distance. For example, reverberations (q.v.) are artefacts. Some artefacts may be helpful in interpreting the image, but others can be very misleading.

Attenuation The decrease in the intensity of the ultrasound waves as they pass through tissues, measured in decibels per centimetre. Attenuation results from absorption, reflection, scattering and beam divergence. In most tissues the attenuation increases approximately linearly with the frequency of the ultrasound.

Axial scan   *See* Transverse scan.

Back wall effect   A bright echo from the back wall of a cyst, resulting from the low attenuation of the beam by the fluid in the cyst and reflection of the beam by the curved back wall.

Beam, acoustic   *See* Acoustic beam.

Boundary   The line at the periphery of two tissues which propagate ultrasound differently, defined by the zone of echoes at the interface.

Coronal plane   A plane running through the body along the long axis (from head to toe) at right angles to the median plane. To scan in this plane, the transducer is placed on the side of the body pointing across to the other side and is moved parallel to the length of the body. A coronal scan may be obtained with the patient supine, prone, erect or lying on one side.

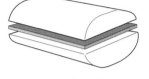

coronal section

Coupling agent   A liquid or gel used to fill the gap between the skin and the ultrasound transducer, so that there is no intervening air to interfere with ultrasound transmission.

Cyst   A fluid-filled structure (mass) with thin walls. A simple cyst characteristically has anechogenic (echo-free) content, with strong back wall reflections and enhancement of the echoes behind the cyst. A cyst can be histologically benign or malignant.

Debris   Echogenic solid masses (of various sizes and shapes, with irregular outlines) within a fluid-filled mass. May be mobile, changing with the patient's position or movement.

Doppler effect   The change in apparent frequency of a wave as a result of relative motion between the observer and the source. The change in frequency is proportional to the speed of motion.

Enhancement, acoustic   *See* Acoustic enhancement.

Focusing   Adjustment of the ultrasound beam so that it converges at a particular depth, in order to improve resolution. Focusing may be electronic or by a lens attached to the transducer.

Frequency   The number of complete ultrasound waves produced each second: for diagnostic ultrasound this is expressed in megahertz. 1 megahertz (MHz) = 10^6 Hz = 10^6 waves per second.

Gain   Amplification of the reflected ultrasound waves by the ultrasound unit. The echoes that come from deep tissues need more amplification than those that come from more superficial tissues, and thus ultrasound units have separate gain controls. The "near gain" control amplifies echoes returning from tissues above the focal point of the beam, while the "far gain" control amplifies echoes returning from tissues beyond the focal point of the beam. These controls can be adjusted to allow proper comparison of echogenicity at different levels.

Hyperechogenic (hyperechoic)

Describes tissues that create brighter echoes than adjacent tissues, e.g. bone, perirenal fat, the wall of the gallbladder, and a cirrhotic liver (compared with normal liver).

Hypoechogenic (hypoechoic)

Describes tissues that create dimmer echoes than adjacent tissues, e.g. lymph nodes, some tumours and fluid. It is important to note that fluid is not the only hypoechogenic material.

Image reversal

Incorrect orientation of the image, i. e. the left side of the image is shown on the right side of the monitor or the positions of the head and feet are reversed. This can be corrected by turning the transducer through 180° or, with some units, electronically. Image reversal is sometimes used to mean a background change, i. e. areas of the image that are normally black are shown as white. This type of image reversal can be corrected electronically.

Impedance, acoustic

See Acoustic impedance.

Interference pattern

Distortion of ultrasound echoes by reflections from other tissues or by the sum of wavelets from adjacent reflectors in a scattering medium, such as liver parenchyma. The result is an artefactual image superimposed on the normal pattern. Such interference can usually be avoided by scanning at different angles.

Internal echoes

Ultrasound reflections from tissues of different density within an organ. Internal echoes may arise from, for example, gallstones within the gallbladder or debris within an abscess.

Lens effect

Narrowing of the ultrasound beam as it passes through certain tissues. The lens effect may sometimes cause a split image.

Longitudinal scan (sagittal scan)

A vertical scan along the long axis of the body. "Sagittal" is usually used to refer to a midline scan, especially in the brain. The landmarks of the midline longitudinal scan include the nose, symphysis pubis and spine. When the scan does not pass through the midline, it may be called "parasagittal". "Longitudinal" is more often used to refer to scans of the abdomen or neck. A longitudinal scan may be obtained with the patient supine, prone, erect or lying on one side.

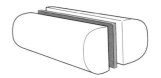

longitudinal section

Mass, complex (mixed mass)

A mass that includes both solid and fluid areas. It will be shown on ultrasound scans as having both echogenic and anechogenic areas; the image will have both non-homogeneous echoes and echo-free spaces (hyper- and hypoechogenic patterns).

Mirror effect   Reflection of all, or nearly all, the ultrasound waves by some tissues or tissue interfaces, e.g. the diaphragm/lung interface. The mirror effect sometimes produces a mirror-image artefact, apparently duplicating the image.

Phantom   A device used for testing and calibrating ultrasound equipment. It has the same range of densities as body tissues. The phantom "tissue" usually contains string and other objects of known reflectivity in known locations.

Reflection   Change in direction of the ultrasound waves at a tissue interface such that the beam does not enter the second tissue. Also known as echo. *See also* Specular reflector.

Reverberation   Reflection of ultrasound waves back and forth between two strongly reflective surfaces that are parallel or nearly parallel. When this occurs, the echoes are delayed in their return to the transducer, and the resulting image may appear deeper than the surfaces actually are. It may also result in duplication, or even triplication, of the image. For example, reverberations may be seen in the anterior part of a distended bladder, or between parallel muscles in the abdominal wall (see page 37).

Sagittal scan   *See* Longitudinal scan.

Scanning plane   The section of tissue through which the ultrasound beam is passing during the scan, and which will appear on the image.

Scattering   Reflection and refraction of ultrasound in many directions at once. This is caused by reflectors whose width is smaller than the wavelength of the ultrasound. Only a small fraction of the transmitted energy is returned to the transducer.

Shadowing, acoustic   *See* Acoustic shadowing.

Solid   Describes tissue that does not include fluid or empty spaces, e.g. solid tumour, liver, muscle, or renal cortex. There will be multiple internal echoes and moderate attenuation of the ultrasound beam.

Specular reflector   Reflective tissue that is smooth and large in comparison with the ultrasound wavelength, e. g. the walls of vessels or tissue membranes. Depending on the angle at which the ultrasound beam meets the reflector, it can reflect all or part of the beam.

Transducer

The part of the ultrasound unit that comes into contact with the patient. It converts electrical energy into ultrasound waves, which pass through the patient's tissues; it also receives the reflected waves and changes them again into electrical energy. A transducer is often called a probe and is connected to the ultrasound scanner (generator and monitor) by a flexible cable. Transducers are expensive and fragile, and must be handled very carefully.

Transverse scan (axial scan)

An ultrasound scan at right angles to the long axis of the body. "Axial" is usually used to refer to scans of the brain, and "transverse" to scans of the abdomen or neck. The beam may be perpendicular or slightly angled to the head or feet of the patient. A transverse scan may be obtained with the patient supine, prone, erect or lying on one side.

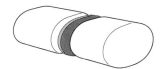

transverse section

Wavelength

The length of a single cycle of the ultrasound wave. It is inversely proportional to the frequency and determines the resolution of the scanner.

Window, acoustic

See Acoustic window.

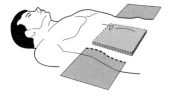

Coronal section

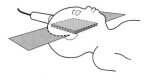

Neonatal coronal section

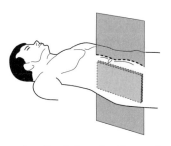

Longitudinal (sagittal) section

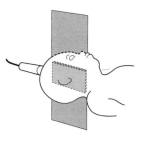

Neonatal sagittal (longitudinal) section

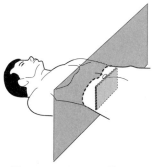

Transverse section

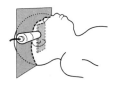

Neonatal axial (transverse) section

Notes

CHAPTER 1

Basics of ultrasound

What is ultrasound?

Ultrasound is the name given to high-frequency sound waves, over 20 000 cycles per second (20 kHz). These waves, inaudible to humans, can be transmitted in beams and are used to scan the tissues of the body.

Ultrasound pulses of the type produced by the scanners described here are of a frequency from 2 to 10 MHz (1 MHz is 1 000 000 cycles per second). The duration of the pulse is about 1 microsecond (a millionth of a second) and the pulses are repeated about 1000 times per second. Different tissues alter the waves in different ways: some reflect directly while others scatter the waves before they return to the transducer as echoes. The waves pass through the tissues at different speeds (for example, 1540 metres per second through soft tissues).

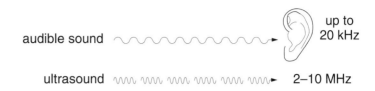

The frequency of ultrasound is many times greater than that of audible sound.

The reflected ultrasound pulses detected by the transducer need to be amplified in the scanner. The echoes that come from deep within the body are more attenuated than those from the more superficial parts, and therefore require more amplification. Ultrasound scanners have controls that can alter the overall sensitivity, the "threshold", of the instrument, as well as change the amplification of the echoes from different depths. When working with any scanner it is necessary to achieve a balanced image, one that contains echoes of approximately equal strengths from all depths of tissue.

When the echoes return to the transducer, it is possible to reconstruct a two-dimensional map of all the tissues that have been in the beams. The information is stored in a computer and displayed on a video (television) monitor. Strong echoes are said to be of "high intensity" and appear as brighter dots on the screen.

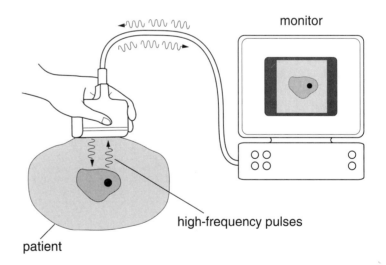

This manual refers only to ultrasound used for medical diagnosis, and not to ultrasound used for other purposes: these require quite different equipment.

Ultrasound generators

The ultrasound waves are generated by a piezoelectric transducer which is capable of changing electrical signals into mechanical (ultrasound) waves. The same transducer can also receive the reflected ultrasound and change it back into electrical signals. Transducers are both transmitters and receivers of ultrasound.

Different modes of ultrasound

The various modes show the returning echoes in different ways.

1. **A-mode**. With this type of ultrasound unit, the echoes are shown as peaks, and the distances between the various structures can be measured (Fig. 1a). This pattern is not usually displayed but similar information is used to build the two-dimensional B-mode image.

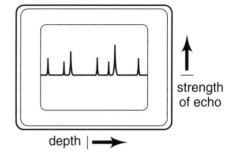

strength of echo

depth |⟶

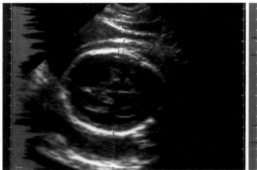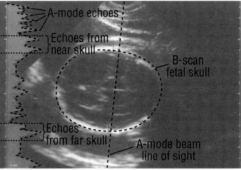

A-mode echoes

Echoes from near skull

B-scan fetal skull

Echoes from far skull

A-mode beam line of sight

Fig. 1a. A-mode scan: the position of the peaks shows the depth of the reflecting structure. The height indicates the strength of the echoes.

2. **B-mode**. This type of image shows all the tissue traversed by the ultrasound scan. The images are two-dimensional and are known as B-mode images or B-mode sections (Fig. 1b). If multiple B-mode images are watched in rapid sequence, they become real-time images.

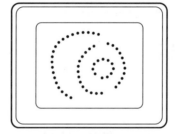

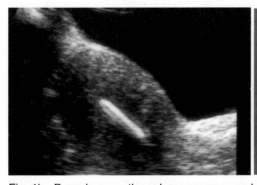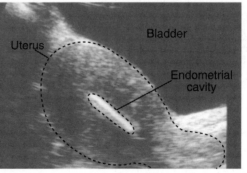

Bladder

Uterus

Endometrial cavity

Fig. 1b. B-mode scan: the echoes are seen as bright dots which show the position of the reflecting structure on a two-dimensional image.

3. **Real-time**. This mode displays motion by showing the images of the part of the body under the transducer as it is being scanned. The images change with each movement of the transducer or if any part of the body is moving (for example, a moving fetus or pulsating artery). The movement is shown on the monitor in real time, as it occurs. In most real-time units, it is possible to "freeze" the displayed image, holding it stationary so that it can be studied and measured if necessary.

4. **M-mode** is another way of displaying motion. The result is a wavy line. This mode is most commonly used for cardiac ultrasound (Fig. 1c).

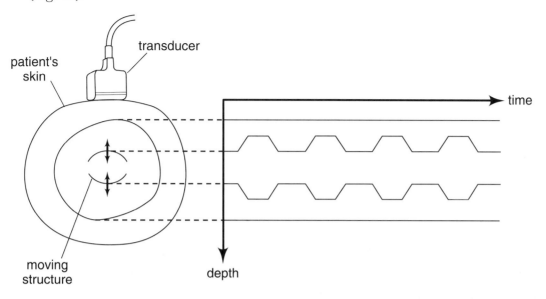

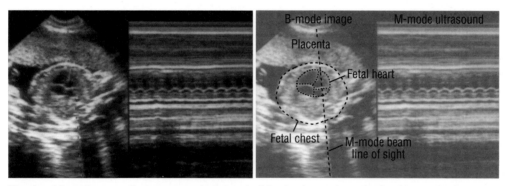

Fig. 1c. M-mode scan: the movement of a part of the body, such as the fetal heart, is shown as a function of time.

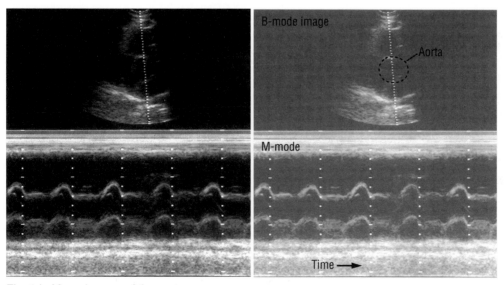

Fig. 1d. M-mode scan of the aorta.

Doppler ultrasound

The electronic circuits for Doppler ultrasound are not included in the general purpose ultrasound specifications. They can be obtained as an inexpensive separate unit, but before deciding to do so, read this section and consider whether the purchase can be justified by the number of patients with treatable vascular disease who are likely to benefit.

> **Do you need Doppler? Read and consider carefully. Is the expense justified?**

The Doppler effect

When ultrasound is transmitted towards a stationary reflector, the reflected waves (echoes) will be of the same frequency as those originally transmitted. However, if the reflector is moving towards the transmitter, the reflected frequency will be higher than the transmitted frequency. Conversely, if the reflector is moving away from the transmitter, the reflected frequency will be lower than the transmitted frequency.

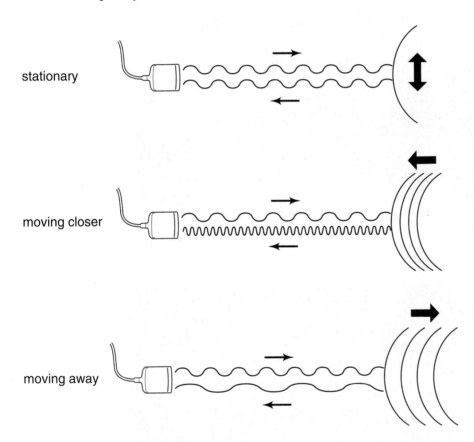

stationary

moving closer

moving away

The difference between the transmitted and received frequencies is proportional to the speed with which the reflector is moving away from or approaching the transmitter. This phenomenon is called the Doppler effect and the difference between the frequencies is called the Doppler shift.

> **Movement *towards* the transducer *increases* the reflected frequency.**

Clinical applications of a Doppler unit

Although an inexpensive Doppler unit can be used to detect fetal heart motion, it is seen better by real-time ultrasound. Doppler can be used to demonstrate blood flow in the peripheral vessels of adults, but in many countries, the number of patients requiring this examination will be relatively few and the additional expense cannot be justified as part of a general purpose ultrasound unit.

The Doppler effect makes it possible to detect and measure the rate of movement of any fluid such as blood. In blood, the moving reflectors are the red blood cells. To measure this movement there are two basic types of Doppler ultrasound unit, the continuous wave (CW) and the pulse wave (PW).

1. **In a continuous wave Doppler unit**, the ultrasound is continuous and the unit measures high velocities accurately, but there is no depth resolution so that all the movement along the ultrasound beam is shown together.

2. **In a pulsed wave Doppler unit**, the ultrasound is transmitted in pulses of ultrasound into the body, with good depth resolution. It can be aimed directly to measure the speed of the blood in a particular vessel (Fig. 2a). The disadvantage is that it cannot measure high blood velocities in deep vessels and high velocities may be wrongly displayed as low velocities (aliasing) (Fig. 2b).

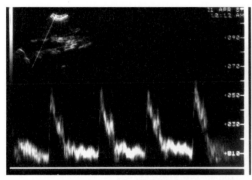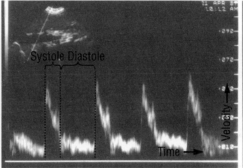

Fig. 2a. Pulsed Doppler scan showing the flow of blood just above the bifurcation of the aorta.

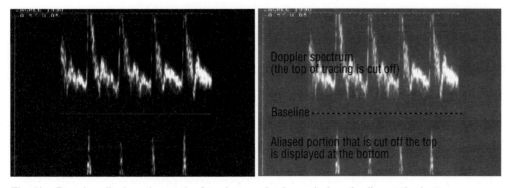

Fig. 2b. Doppler aliasing: the peak of each wave is shown below the line at the bottom, indicating negative flow. These aliasing artefacts occur when the pulse repetition rate of the unit is not sufficiently high to measure the high velocity of the reflecting structure.

3. **In a colour Doppler unit** (a further development on the above principle), the distribution and direction of the flowing blood are shown as a two-dimensional image in which the velocities are distinguished by different colours.

4. **In a duplex Doppler system**, a blood vessel is located by B-mode ultrasound imaging and then the blood flow is measured by Doppler ultrasound. This combination of a B-mode and Doppler system allows the Doppler beam to be directed more accurately at any particular blood vessel (Fig. 2c,d).

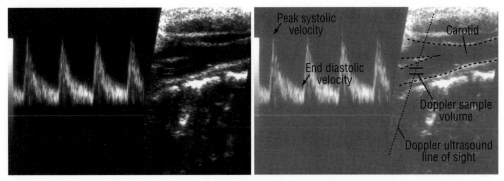

Fig. 2c. Duplex Doppler image of the internal carotid artery. On the left is the Doppler shift spectrum indicating pulsatile flow towards the transducer. If the flow was away from the transducer, the spectrum would be upside down. The line is wavy, because the blood velocity changes during the heart cycle. On the right is a B-mode image showing where the blood flow is being recorded.

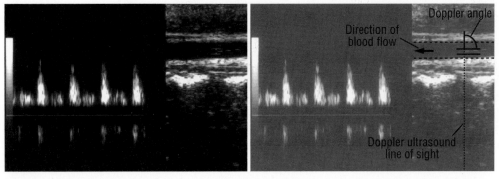

Fig. 2d. If the scanning angle is not correct, the result can be misleading. This is the common carotid artery of the patient shown in Fig. 2c, but scanned at an angle of nearly 90°. As a result, the flow appears disturbed, while it was, in fact, quite normal. The angle is wrong, not the blood flow.

Wave propagation

Wave propagation describes the transmission and spread of ultrasound waves to different tissues. The differences in the ways in which ultrasound interacts with tissues influence the design of an ultrasound unit, affect the interpretation of the images and impose limitations on the usefulness of the method.

Ultrasound waves propagate as longitudinal waves in soft tissues. The molecules vibrate and deliver energy to each other so that ultrasound energy propagates through the body. The average propagation speed for soft tissues is 1540 metres per second.

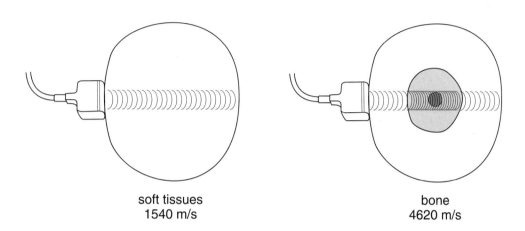

soft tissues
1540 m/s

bone
4620 m/s

Wavelength

The wavelength of ultrasound is inversely proportional to its frequency. The higher the frequency, the shorter the wavelength. For example, ultrasound of 3 MHz has a wavelength of 0.5 mm in soft tissue, whereas ultrasound of 6 MHz has a wavelength of 0.25 mm. The shorter the wavelength, the better the resolution, giving a clearer image and more details on the screen. However, wavelength also affects the way in which the waves go through the tissues (see "Attenuation", p. 11).

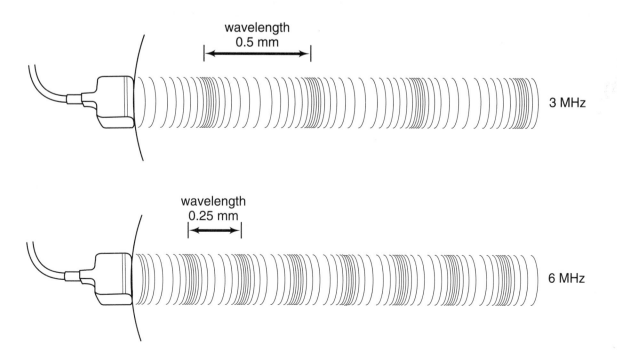

wavelength
0.5 mm

3 MHz

wavelength
0.25 mm

6 MHz

Focusing

Ultrasound waves can be focused either by lenses and mirrors or electronically in composite transducers. In the same way that a thin beam of light shows an object more clearly than a widely scattered, unfocused beam, so with focused ultrasound: a narrow beam images a thin section of tissue and thus gives better detail. For best results it is necessary to focus at the depth in the body that is of most relevance to the particular clinical problem. For general purpose scanners this usually means using different transducers for different purposes and adjusting the focal zone on the unit as necessary (Fig. 3).

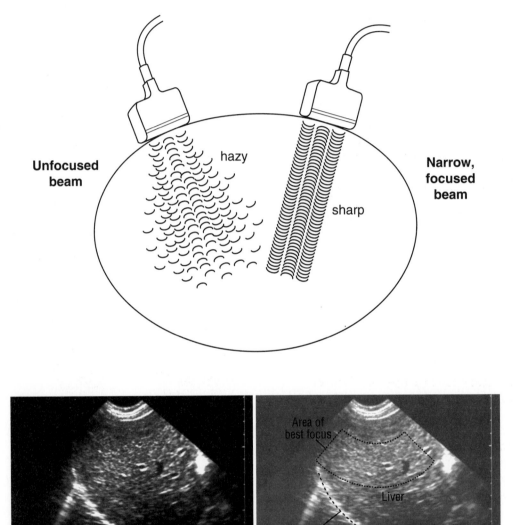

Fig. 3. The centre of this image is in focus, while the periphery is not.

Variable focus

Many transducers have a fixed focus. Composite transducers, such as a linear and convex array, and annular sector transducers (see pp. 14–15) have an electronically variable focal length which can be adjusted to the required depth. However, most transducers have a fixed focal distance in at least one plane: only annular array sector transducers have an adjustable electronic focus in all planes. Well adjusted focusing provides a narrow acoustic beam and a thinner image section: this gives better resolution of details and a clearer picture with more information.

Attenuation

Tissues in the body absorb and scatter ultrasound in different ways. Higher frequencies are more readily absorbed and scattered (attenuated) than lower frequencies. Thus, to reach deeper tissues, it is necessary to use lower frequencies because the waves are less likely to be diverted as they traverse intervening structures. In practice, it is better to use about 3.5 MHz for deep scanning in adults and 5 MHz or higher if available for scanning the thinner bodies of children. 5 MHz or greater is also best for scanning superficial organs in adults.

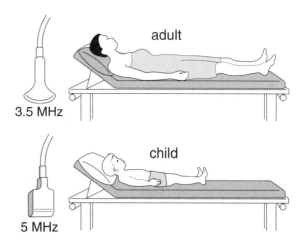

adult

3.5 MHz

child

5 MHz

Higher frequency shows more details but is less penetrating.

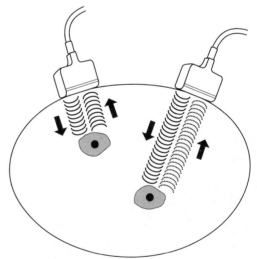

5 MHz

3.5 MHz

High frequencies have better resolution but less depth.

Low frequencies penetrate better but have less resolution.

Amplification

The echoes that return from deeper structures are not as strong as those that come from tissues nearer the surface; they must, therefore, be amplified and in the ultrasound unit this is done by the time-gain-compensation (TGC) amplifier. In all ultrasound units it is possible to vary the degree of amplification to compensate for ultrasound attenuation in any part of the body and improve the quality of the final image (Fig. 4).

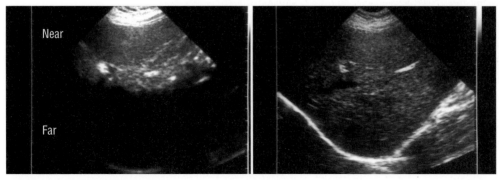

Near

Far

Fig. 4. On the left the far gain is too low and no echoes have returned from the deeper tissues. On the right the gain has been corrected and the returning echoes are of equal strength throughout.

Boundaries

Ultrasound may be reflected or refracted (bent) when it meets the boundary between two different types of tissue: reflection means the waves are thrown back and refraction means they change in direction and are not necessarily reflected (see also p. 13 and p. 27).

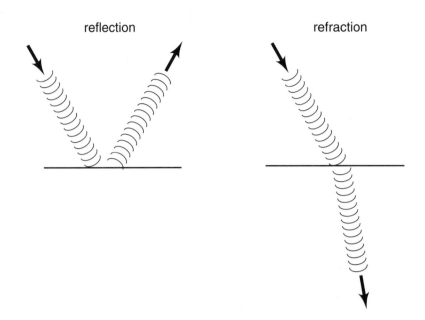

Tissues vary greatly in their effect on ultrasound. For example, the skeleton and gas in the bowel or chest behave very differently from soft tissue. When ultrasound waves meet bone or gas in the body, they are significantly reflected and refracted. Thus, it is usually impossible to use ultrasound effectively when there is a lot of gas in the bowel: when examining the pelvis the urinary bladder should be as full as possible to lift the intestine out of the way. Because of the effect of air, the normal lungs cannot be examined at all by ultrasound, but pleural fluid or a mass in contact with the chest wall can be imaged.

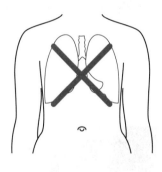

The skeleton reflects ultrasound so strongly that the architecture within a bone or heavily calcified tissue cannot be seen and there is an acoustic shadow behind it. As a result, imaging through an adult skull or other bones is not possible (Fig. 5) (see p. 35).

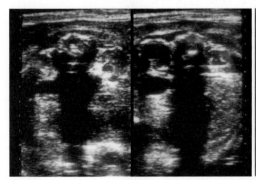
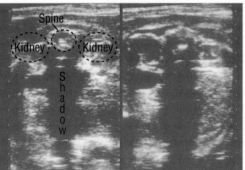

Fig. 5. Two transverse scans through a fetus. showing shadows caused by the fetal spine. Similar shadows below ribs may obscure parts of the kidneys or liver. Changing the angle of a scan will alter the position of a shadow so that underlying tissues can be seen clearly (see p. 28).

A fraction of the incident wave (1) is reflected (2) at an angle equal to the angle of incidence. Another fraction (3) passes across the interface and is refracted, continuing at an angle that is different from the angle of incidence. The greater the difference between the characteristic acoustic impedances, the greater the fraction which is reflected. The greater the ratio of the propagation speeds, the greater the refraction. In practice, this is most important when the incident angle is zero and the ultrasound wave strikes the interface perpendicularly.

If the reflecting boundary is much wider than the wavelength (e.g. 10 or 20 times wider), it acts like a mirror and is called a specular reflector.

The fetal skull, the diaphragm, the walls of vessels and the connective tissues are examples of specular reflectors (Fig. 6).

Ultrasound waves scatter when the width of the reflectors (scatterers) is smaller than the wavelength of the ultrasound. Only a small fraction of the ultrasound wave is scattered back in the original direction.

The liver and the kidney parenchyma are examples of scattering media.

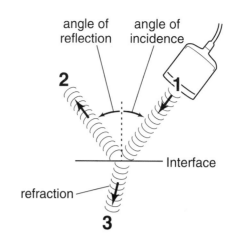

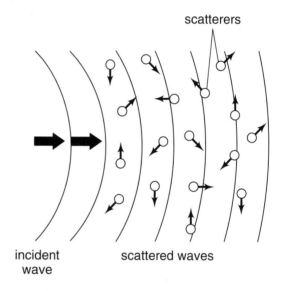

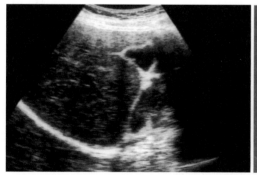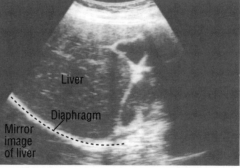

Fig. 6. Sagittal liver scan: there is strong (specular) reflection from the diaphragm, which is such a strong reflector that the image of the liver is repeated behind it. The ultrasound waves travel across the liver first at transmission, again after being reflected from the diaphragm, then again from the tissue interfaces.

It is because of boundary effects that a coupling agent must be used for scanning, to prevent air trapped between the skin and the transducer acting as a barrier to the ultrasound waves.

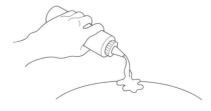

Transducers (scanning probes)

The transducer is the most expensive part of any ultrasound unit. The probe contains one or more transducers that transmit the ultrasound pulses and receive back the echoes during scanning. Each transducer is focused at a particular depth. The beam of ultrasound emitted varies in shape and size depending on the type of transducer and the generator.

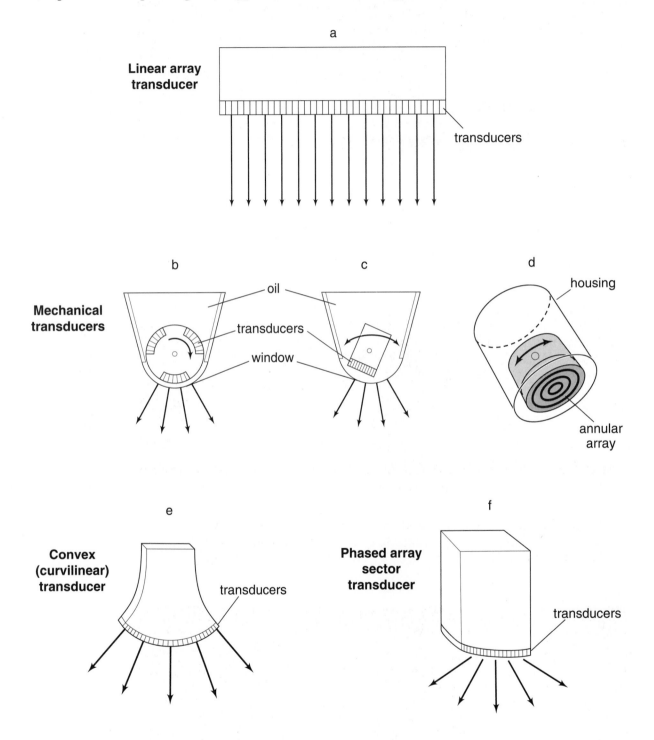

The shape of the scans from different transducers

1. **Linear array**. Scans from this type of transducer are rectangular. They are most useful in obstetrics and for scanning the breast and the thyroid (Fig. 7a).

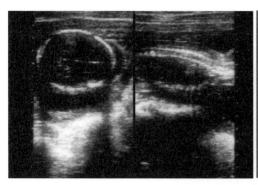
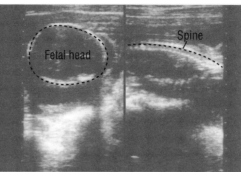
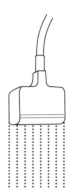

Fig. 7a. The rectangular image from a linear array transducer.

2. **Sector scanner**. These scans are fan-shaped, almost triangular, and originate through a very small acoustic window. These scanners can be used whenever there is only a small space available for scanning. They are most useful in the upper abdomen and for gynaecological and cardiological examinations (Fig. 7b).

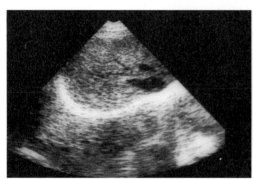
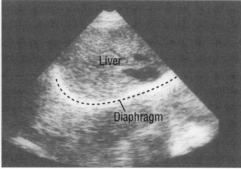
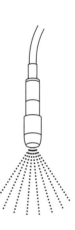

Fig. 7b. The fan-shaped image from a sector transducer.

3. **Convex transducer**. This produces a scan somewhere between those of the linear and the sector scanners and is therefore useful for all parts of the body except for specialized echocardiography Fig. 7c).

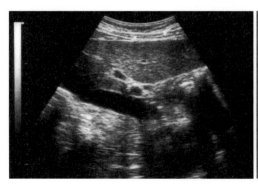
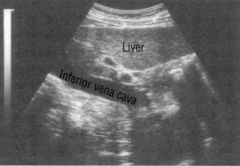
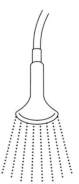

Fig. 7c. The wide fan-shaped image with a broad, curved apex from a convex transducer.

Summary

A-mode:	**peaks and distances. Not often used.**
B-mode:	**two-dimensional images in which the echo amplitude is depicted as dots of different brightness.**
Real time:	**shows movement as it occurs.**
M-mode:	**shows movement as a function of time. Used in cardiac scanning.**
Doppler:	**demonstrates and measures blood flow.**
Colour Doppler:	**shows different flow-velocities in different colours.**

CHAPTER 2

Choosing an ultrasound scanner

Choose a scanner that will perform the examinations needed at your hospital; there is no justification for buying accessories or gadgets that are not likely to be used very often. The scanner should at least match the specifications given in the Annex (p. 321). Apart from the technical specifications, there are some basic rules to be observed when choosing a scanner.

The monitor

The monitor (viewing screen) should be at least 13 cm × 10 cm (or about 16 cm diagonally).

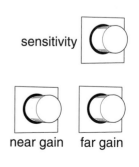

The scanner

1. The scanner should be portable and light enough to be carried by hand for 100 metres.

2. The scanner must be suitable for use in the local climate, i.e. protected from dust or capable of being used in high or low temperatures, as appropriate.

3. The scanner must be tough enough to withstand adverse transport and storage conditions. It should not be damaged by movement in an aircraft or in a vehicle on rough roads.

4. The scanner must operate satisfactorily from the power supply in the hospital or clinic where it is going to be used. This requirement should be checked and double-checked before the scanner is accepted. The unit should be compatible with local voltage and frequency, and it should be able to stabilize fluctuations in supply.

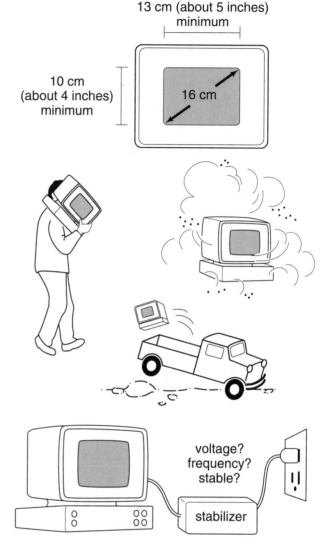

Servicing the scanner

Servicing must be available within a reasonable distance. It may be wise to purchase a unit similar to other scanners in use in the area, so that sufficient expertise and spare parts are available.

What controls are needed on the scanner?

The scanner must be equipped with a video monitor (TV screen) and to control the images there must be:

1. An overall sensitivity control to alter the amount of information on the video screen.

2. Separate controls to alter the surface (near) echoes and the deep (distant) echoes. These are known as near gain and far gain controls.

3. A control (frame freeze) to hold the image on the screen so that it can be viewed for as long as necessary.

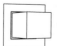

4. A control to measure the distance between two points shown on the image. This should be done electronically and usually means positioning a small dot at each end of the length to be measured. The distance between the dots should be shown automatically in centimetres or millimetres on the screen. Biometric tables (for obstetrics) are an advantage.

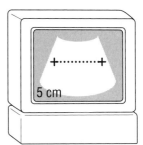

Recording the image

It should be possible to add patient identification and other data to the image electronically: it is very desirable that a permanent record of important scans be put in the patient's medical record. There are several ways to do this, varying in cost and efficiency.

1. The best and most expensive method is to record the image on an X-ray film. This requires an image-processing unit and a special camera. It may be necessary to have a darkroom. Ordinary X-ray film can be used but the best results are obtained using single-emulsion X-ray film, which is expensive. Prints on paper are less expensive but not always of the same quality (see item 3, below).

2. The next best method is also expensive: it requires a self-processing camera and film specifically designed to be attached to the ultrasound unit. Both the camera and the films are expensive and films are not always readily available. However, the results are good and the prints can be seen almost immediately.

3. There are image-recording units that will print the image on special paper (this is much less expensive than using film). The images are quite satisfactory for routine records, but the paper must be protected from excessive heat and light.

4. The image on the screen can be photographed on black and white film using most 35 mm reflex cameras. An additional close-up lens may be necessary. The film will then have to be processed and printed in the usual way. This can take time, especially in a rural hospital.

5. If it is not possible to purchase any type of recording unit, exact details of the findings and relevant measurements must be noted in the patient's record at the time of the scan.

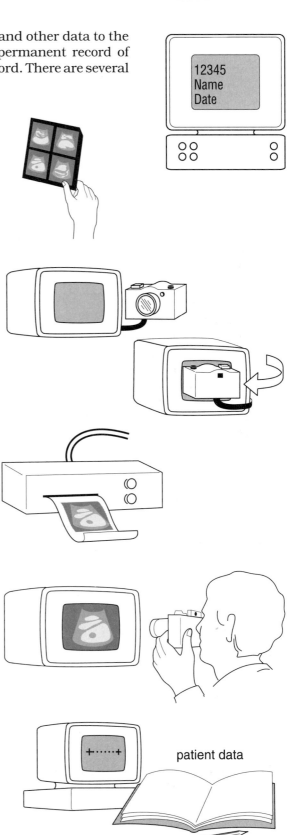

patient data

Nothing must be left to memory.

Choosing the appropriate transducer

The best transducer for general work is a convex transducer of 3.5 MHz focused at 7–9 cm. If this type of transducer is not available then both linear and sector transducers of 3.5 MHz will be necessary. If children or thin adults are to be scanned, an additional 5.0 MHz transducer focused at 5–7 cm is helpful.

1. **Obstetric ultrasound**. If most of the ultrasound examinations will be for general obstetrics, the transducer should be linear or convex, either 3.5 or 5.0 MHz focused at 7–9 cm. If only one transducer can be purchased, choose 3.5 MHz. The 5 MHz transducer is best during early pregnancy: the 3.5 MHz is better in later pregnancy.

2. **General purpose ultrasound.** If the examinations will include the upper abdomen of adults and the pelvis, as well as obstetrics, a sector or convex transducer of 3.5 MHz focused at 7–9 cm is most suitable.

3. **Paediatric ultrasound.** For children a 5.0 MHz transducer with a focus of about 5–7 cm is needed. If neonatal brain scans are to be carried out, a sector transducer of 7.5 MHz focused at 4–5 cm will be required (and can be helpful for adult testis and neck).

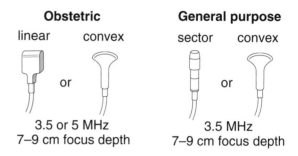

Obstetric

linear   convex

or

3.5 or 5 MHz
7–9 cm focus depth

General purpose

sector   convex

or

3.5 MHz
7–9 cm focus depth

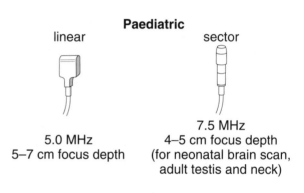

Paediatric

linear   sector

5.0 MHz
5–7 cm focus depth

7.5 MHz
4–5 cm focus depth
(for neonatal brain scan,
adult testis and neck)

Summary

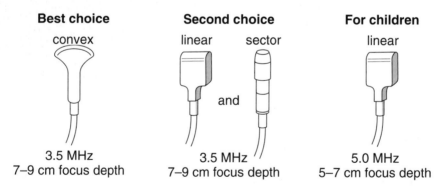

Best choice

convex

3.5 MHz
7–9 cm focus depth

Second choice

linear   sector

and

3.5 MHz
7–9 cm focus depth

For children

linear

5.0 MHz
5–7 cm focus depth

The complete ultrasound unit

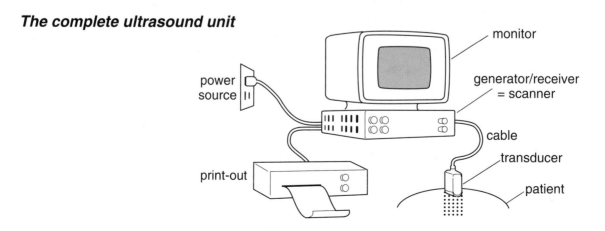

What is needed in the ultrasound scanning room?

No radiation protection is needed.

There is no dangerous radiation from a medical diagnostic ultrasound machine and walls of any material are satisfactory. However, the room must be kept dry and free from dust.

The room must be big enough to accommodate the scanner, a couch, a chair and a small table or desk. It should be large enough to allow a trolley to be wheeled in and the patient to be transferred to the couch. There must be a door to ensure privacy.

The couch should be firm but soft, and it should be possible to lift one end so that the patient can recline comfortably. If the couch is on wheels there must be good brakes. Two firm pillows should be available. The couch should be easy to clean.

There should be facilities for washing hands and providing drinking-water, preferably in the room, and there should be a toilet nearby.

There must be a window or some other form of ventilation and adequate lighting, preferably with a dimmer switch or some other way of varying the brightness of the lights. Bright sunlight should be screened or curtained off. If the room is too bright, it will not be easy to see the images on the video screen.

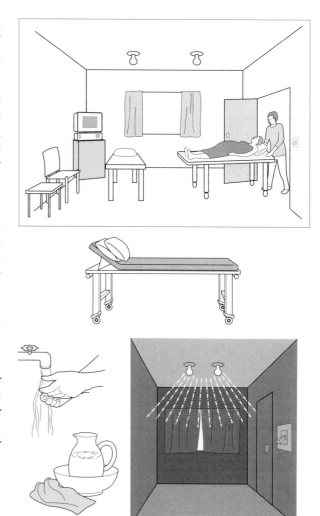

What electrical outlets are needed?

No special electrical power supply is required: a standard wall outlet is all that is usually necessary, for example, 220 V at 5 A or 110 V at 10 A. No special electrical connection is needed but the exact specifications of the equipment should be verified with the supplier. It is important that the ultrasound unit to be purchased is suitable for use with the available electrical supply and the company that sells the equipment should be required to check and confirm this in writing.

The main electrical supply to many hospitals or clinics, particularly in the developing world, is very variable in both voltage and frequency. If there is too much fluctuation, the ultrasound unit may be damaged or, at the very least, function poorly. It may be necessary to buy a good voltage stabilizer. This should be determined before the equipment is purchased.

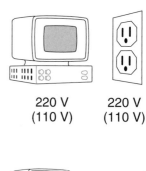

220 V   220 V
(110 V)   (110 V)

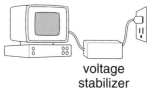

voltage
stabilizer

When the scanner is delivered

It is important to check every aspect of the scanner before the person who delivers the equipment has left. Whatever is happening, take time to do this because once he or she has gone, it may be too late!

Every new ultrasound unit must be supplied with a detailed user's manual and a service manual, either separate or combined. Make sure that they are there when the unit is delivered and are complete, particularly if supplied in a loose-leaf binder.

Open the user's manual and look at the instructions. Go through them, checking the controls one by one as described in the manual: make sure you can follow the instructions.

service manual

user's manual

Check every instruction in the manual. Taking time to do this may save a lot of money and frustration!

It is *not* sufficient to watch the supplier demonstrate the unit upon delivery.

Try all the controls and every aspect of the equipment for yourself.

Use the following as a checklist:

1. Confirm that the plugs provided will fit into the outlets of the electrical supply.

2. Confirm that the voltage setting for the unit is compatible with the electrical supply.

3. Turn on the unit and make sure there is no interference on the screen. (If the electrical supply also powers an air-conditioner, surgical diathermy, a faulty fluorescent-tube starter or other electrical equipment, artefacts may appear on the screen.) Test the unit on a patient or colleague. Check all the controls individually.

4. The operation of all transducers and their cables can be tested by slowly moving a pencil, lubricated with coupling agent, along the transducer surface. The image should not disappear from the monitor while the pencil is in contact with any part of the transducer in any position. (Repeat this examination with the transducer above, alongside and under the pencil or test object.) Make sure that movement of the cable which connects the transducer to the ultrasound unit does not cause any blurring, loss of clarity or change in the image (see opposite).

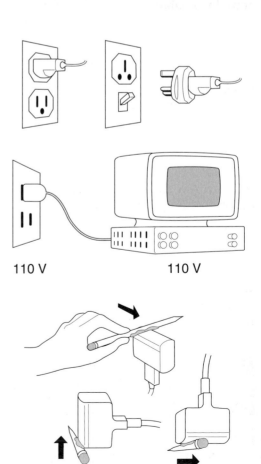

110 V 110 V

5. A sector transducer can be tested by scanning a hypodermic needle through the side or bottom of a beaker full of water. The image of the needle should not move if the needle is kept still.

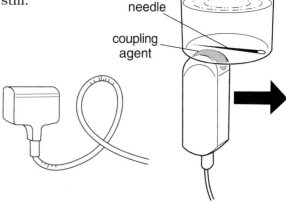

6. Bending the cable while the transducer is held in position should not cause any change, and certainly no movement or blurring, of the image.

7. Check any electronic method of measuring length and make sure the electronic pointers are clearly seen on the screen and that distances can be easily read.

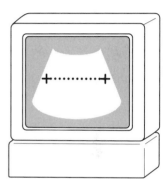

8. If the unit is provided with automatic biometric or measurement tables, try out all of them to make sure the stored data are readily accessible and easily read.

9. All biometric measurements or tables that are programmed into the unit should be tested to make sure that all the data specified are actually available on the equipment.

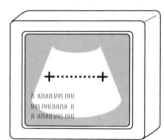

10. Check that the service and maintenance manual is available and complete.

11. Receive and check a fully completed and dated written guarantee (warranty).

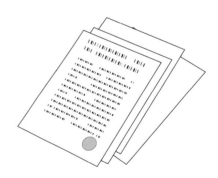

12. Withhold the final payment for the equipment until it has been used for one month and is working satisfactorily.

Learn to use ultrasound by scanning normal people (this is quite safe) with this manual beside you. With time and practice, you should be able to recognize on the video screen the normal images shown in this manual and identify all the anatomical landmarks.

Notes

CHAPTER 3

Basic rules of scanning

Orientation of the image

It is possible for the images on the monitor to be reversed so that, on transverse scans, the left side of the patient is seen on the right side of the screen. Although there may be an indicator on the transducer, it is essential before scanning to check visually which side of the transducer produces which side of the image. This is best done by putting a finger at one end of the transducer and seeing where it appears on the screen. If incorrect, rotate the transducer 180° and check again (Fig. 8a). On longitudinal scans, the head of the patient should be on the left side and the feet on the right side of the screen.

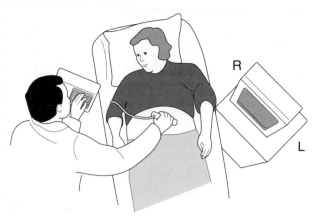

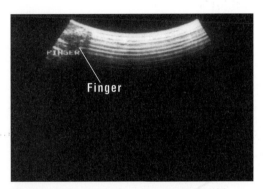

Fig. 8a. A finger on the transducer should produce an image on the same side of the screen. If the image is on the wrong side, rotate the transducer by 180°.

Incorrect　　　　**Correct**

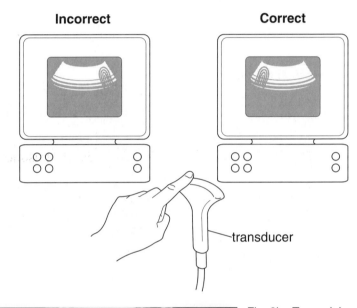

transducer

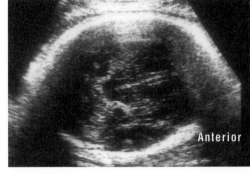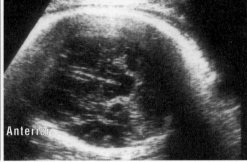

Fig. 8b. Two axial images of the same fetal head, but aligned 180° differently. When starting to scan, the images on the screen must be tested as shown in Fig. 8a.

Contact with the patient's skin

The transducer must be moved across the patient; therefore, the patient's skin in the region to be examined must always be amply covered with a coupling agent (see pp. 44–45) to allow transmission of the ultrasound beam and easy movement of the transducer.

While the transducer is moved slowly across the patient it must always be kept in close contact with the skin through the coupling agent; movement must be continuous and gradual while the operator carefully watches the image on the screen.

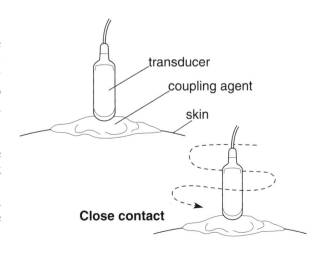

transducer

coupling agent

skin

Close contact

Background of the image

The image on the screen may be predominantly black or predominantly white. It may have a white background with black echoes (Fig. 9 upper), or a black background with white echoes showing as spots or lines (Fig. 9 lower). There is usually a switch to make this change; if not, an engineer should adjust the machine so that it always shows a *black background with white echoes* (Fig. 9 lower).

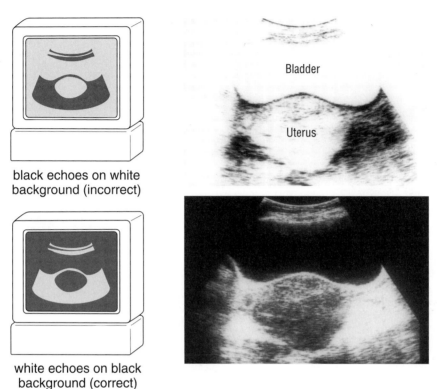

black echoes on white background (incorrect)

white echoes on black background (correct)

Bladder

Uterus

Fig. 9. Transverse images of an enlarged uterus with the background changed.

Distribution of the ultrasound beam

Body tissues reflect ultrasound in two different ways. Some tissues act like mirrors, sending the waves directly back. Others scatter the waves in the way fog scatters a beam of light. For example, the diaphragm is a "mirror", known technically as a "specular reflector". The monitor will show a clear and exact image that corresponds well with the position and the shape of the diaphragm. The liver, however, scatters ultrasound waves and the position of the dots shown on the screen does not exactly correspond with any particular detail in the liver. This is an "interference pattern" resulting from waves being scattered in different directions. In either case, the use of a black background with white echoes permits better differentiation.

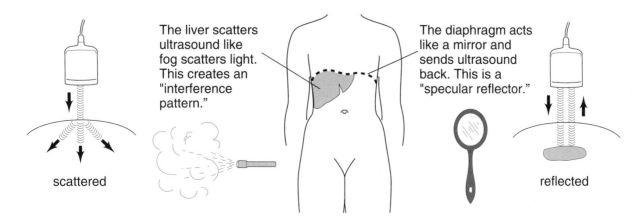

scattered

The liver scatters ultrasound like fog scatters light. This creates an "interference pattern."

The diaphragm acts like a mirror and sends ultrasound back. This is a "specular reflector."

reflected

Acoustic enhancement and shadowing

Clear liquids allow ultrasound to pass directly through without much alteration, so that echoes that come from tissue behind liquid are usually enhanced (brighter). This is known as "acoustic enhancement" (Fig. 10a). Drinking enough water to fill the stomach will displace gas-filled bowel, providing an acoustic window. This is particularly useful in visualizing the body and tail of the pancreas.

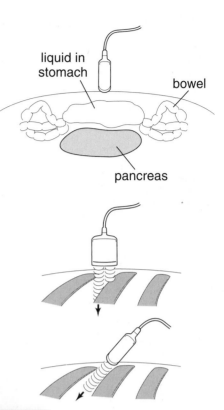

Gas in the bowel or elsewhere can present a variety of sonographic patterns. The beam can be scattered, reflected, absorbed, and refracted, making it very difficult to image underlying structures. For this reason, ultrasound cannot be used to image the normal lungs or to demonstrate lung disease other than peripheral masses. A chest X-ray provides much better information.

Dense materials such as bones or calculi (stones) cast shadows on structures behind them, because the ultrasound waves do not go through them. This is known as "acoustic shadowing". For example, ribs may obstruct the field of view so the structures behind must be examined obliquely through the intercostal spaces (Fig. 10b, c) (see also p. 35).

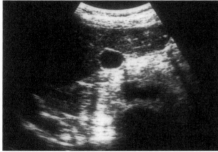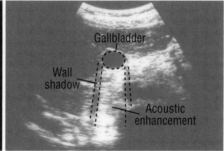

Fig. 10a. A liquid-filled structure, the gallbladder, with posterior enhancement due to low ultrasound attenuation. The walls of the gallbladder cause two lateral shadows.

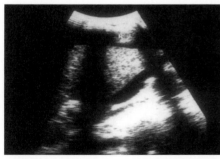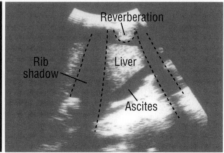

Fig. 10b. When the liver and ascites are imaged through the ribs, the ribs cast two shadows and there is a layer of reverberation in the ascites (see also p. 37).

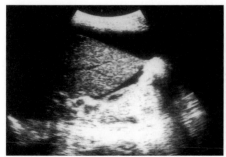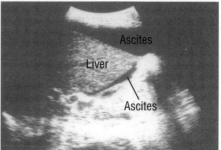

Fig. 10c. Imaging the same patient at an angle through the intercostal space eliminates the rib shadows and the reverberation.

Frequency and resolution

The higher the frequency of the ultrasound, the better the resolution. This means that smaller details become visible when higher frequency is used. However, the penetration of the ultrasound into the body will be less. Scanning is, therefore, a compromise and the highest frequency that is also sufficient to penetrate deeply enough should always be used (Fig. 11) (see also p. 9 and 11).

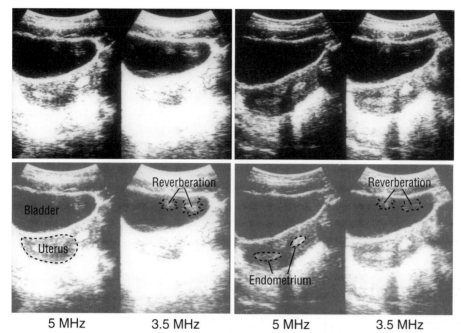

5 MHz   3.5 MHz   5 MHz   3.5 MHz

Fig. 11. Images of a uterus made at different scanner frequencies. Quality is best judged by comparing the details of the endometrium. There is reverberation in the liquid-filled urinary bladder.

Focus of the ultrasound beam

Because the organs or parts of the body that are of interest will be at different depths, the focus of the transducer should ideally be adjustable (pp. 10 and 20). If the focal distance is fixed, the most suitable transducer must be chosen for the particular examination. The best choice is described in each section of the manual.

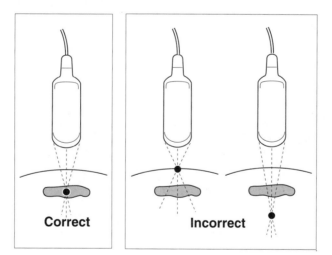

Correct   **Incorrect**

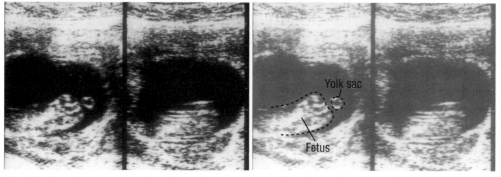

Fig. 12. The focus is correct on the left, showing details of the yolk sac; on the right there are no details because the focus is set too deep.

Sensitivity and gain

It is important to know that the wrong sensitivity (gain) setting can make diagnosis inaccurate or even impossible.

Fig. 13 shows the effect of varying the sensitivity and gain controls.

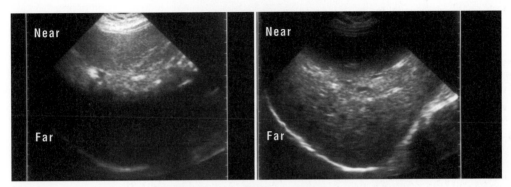

Fig. 13a. Liver ultrasound. Left: low far gain. Right: low near gain.

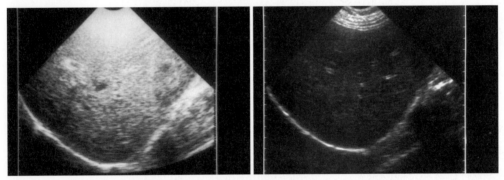

Fig. 13b. Liver ultrasound. Left: high overall gain. Right: low overall gain.

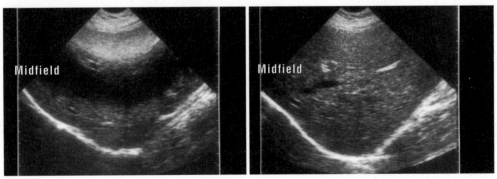

Fig. 13c. Liver ultrasound. Left: low midfield gain. Right: correct gain.

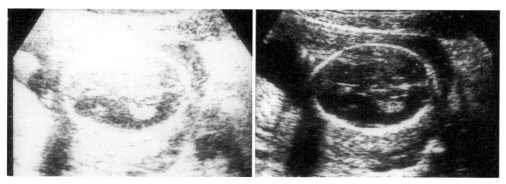

Fig. 13d. Fetal skull. Left: the overall sensitivity is too high. Right: the overall sensitivity is now correct but too high for accurate measurement of the biparietal diameter.

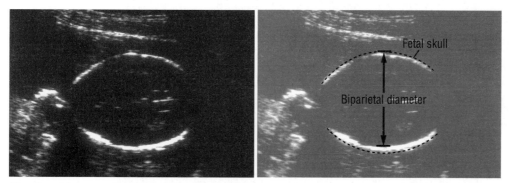

Fig. 13e. The overall sensitivity is now too low for general scanning, but correct for the measurement of the biparietal diameter.

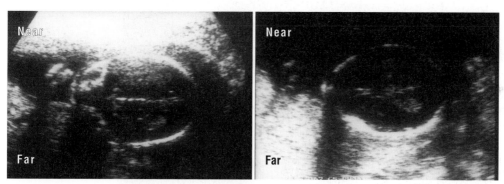

Fig. 13f. Left: poor definition because the near gain is too high; compare the indistinct image of the upper part of the skull with the much clearer lower half (compare Fig. 13d and e; see also p. 33). Right: the gain has been overcorrected; the near gain is now too low and the far gain is too high.

If the image is poor even when the gain has been changed, apply more coupling agent.

Artefacts

An artefact is an additional, missing or distorted image which does not conform to the real image of the part being examined. Artefacts do not arise from the primary ultrasound beam, or direct echoes from the part being scanned, but result from distortion or attenuation of the image. There are many different causes. Recognition of such artefacts is important because they can be misleading and may even be mistaken for some important finding that may affect the diagnosis. Other artefacts may provide important additional information and should be recognized and used.

Cysts

A cyst usually appears as an echo-free area and the structures behind the cyst are enhanced: there are no echoes from within cysts because there are no impedance interfaces within the liquid. Because the liquid does not absorb ultrasound to the same extent as tissue, the echoes from behind the cyst are over-compensated by the equipment and appear enhanced—the strong back wall effect (Fig. 14a, b).

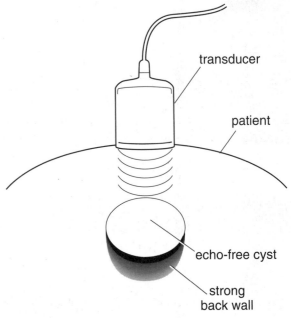

> A cyst is seen as an echo-free area with a strong back wall. If there are echoes within a cyst, these may be real or artefactual.

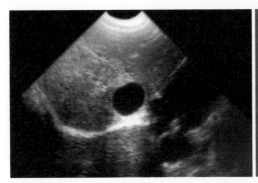
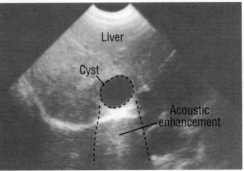

Fig. 14a. A liquid-filled cyst in the liver: there are no internal echoes and there is a strong back wall effect.

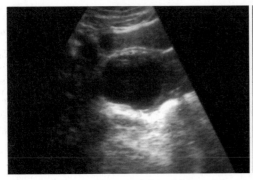
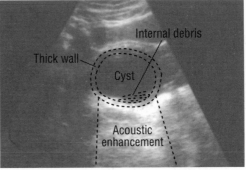

Fig. 14b. This ovarian cyst has thick walls and contains debris. This causes echoes within the cyst, which will probably alter when the patient is scanned in a different position (see pp. 34–35).

If the gain is *too low*, a solid mass may appear cystic without internal echoes. There will be no strong back wall effect (no enhancement).

If the gain is *too high*, a fluid-filled structure may fill with echoes and resemble a solid mass.

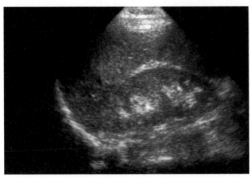
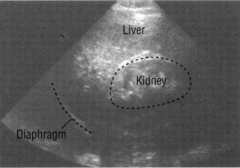

Fig. 14c. Longitudinal scan: the gain is incorrectly adjusted, so that the outline of the kidney and the periphery of the liver are not well seen.

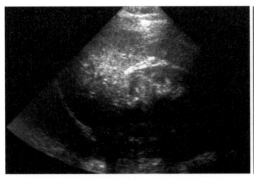
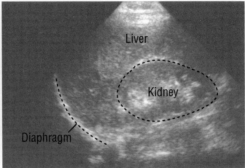

Fig. 14d. Longitudinal scan with proper gain: the margins of the kidney and the internal details of the kidney and liver are now well defined.

Near and far gain must also be carefully adjusted (Fig. 14e–f).

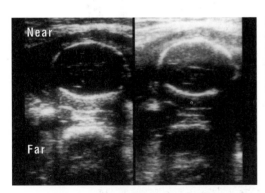

Fig. 14e. Images of the fetal head. Left: balanced image of low sensitivity. Right: near gain too high; it must be reduced while the overall gain is increased to obtain a good image of the whole head.

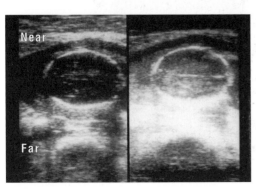

Fig. 14f. Left: a well balanced image. Right: far gain too high, near gain too low; the far gain must be reduced and the near gain increased.

A space, such as a cyst filled with clear fluid, appears to be free of echoes on the screen. The walls of the cyst reflect the ultrasound at an angle so that information does not return to the transducer. This results in acoustic shadows laterally, but behind the cystic area the echoes will be enhanced (the strong back wall) (Fig. 15).

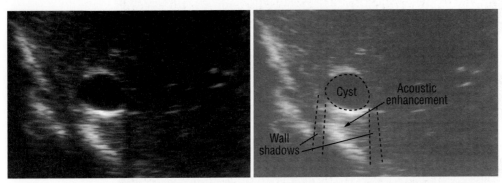

Fig. 15a. A hepatic cyst: the internal fluid is clear, and there are no echoes. The walls of the cyst reflect the ultrasound away from the transducer, causing lateral shadows.

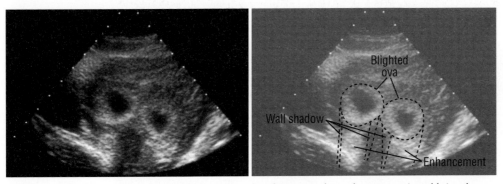

Fig. 15b. Blighted ova: two liquid-filled spaces showing posterior enhancement and lateral shadowing.

Artefacts may be seen in any cystic structure (such as the urinary bladder or gallbladder) and tend to be seen anteriorly, becoming less intense with depth. They may disappear or change in character as the transducer is moved. However, real structures in a cyst, such as septa, maintain their relationships regardless of the position of the transducer. True echoes can be due to reflection from blood clot, pus or necrotic debris, and these tend to be at the bottom of the cyst: if not attached to the wall, they will move when the patient changes position (Fig. 16).

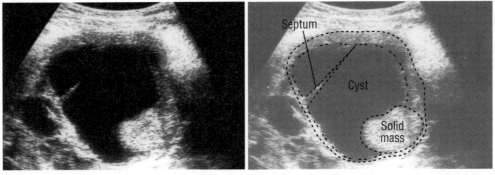

Fig 16a. Malignant ovarian cyst: a large cyst with an internal septum, which did not alter when the patient was scanned in different positions.

Debris within a cyst may float, forming a level which will vary as the patient's position changes (Fig. 16b, c).

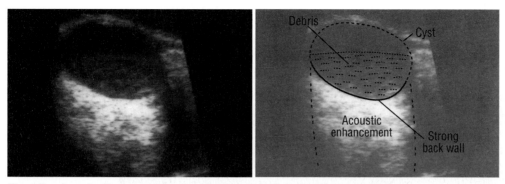

Fig. 16b. A cyst with a strong back wall, lateral shadows and internal debris.

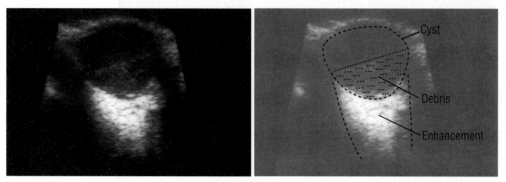

Fig. 16c. The same patient as in Fig. 16b scanned in a different position. The floating debris has moved.

Shadows

Bone, calculi and calcification result in an acoustic shadow. Ultrasound cannot pass through bone unless it is very thin (e.g., the skull of a neonate). In order to see what is behind, a different angle of scanning must be used (Fig. 17a, b).

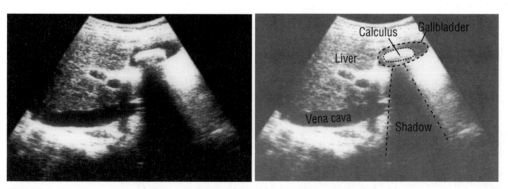

Fig. 17a. A large acoustic shadow below a calculus in the gallbladder.

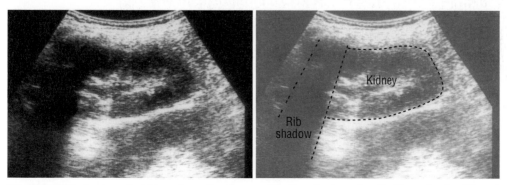

Fig. 17b. This image of a kidney is partly obscured by the shadow of a rib. Scanning in different phases of respiration may move the kidney out of the shadow.

Abdominal wall

Significant subcutaneous fat and muscle can scatter ultrasound, making the images of deeper structures less distinct. Sometimes the muscles cause a double ultrasound image giving a false impression of separation: an incorrect diagnosis (e.g. of twins) may result. Always use multiple projections at different angles to confirm any suspected abnormality (Fig. 18).

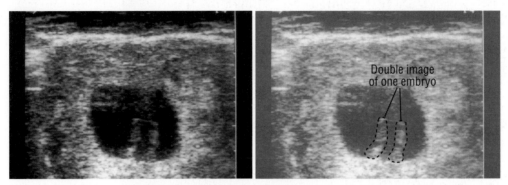

Fig. 18. Muscles, especially the abdominal muscles, can act as convex lenses. This early pregnancy looks like a twin pregnancy because the lens effect of the rectus muscle causes the borders of the gestational sac to be imaged twice. On a longitudinal scan the "twin" could not be found.

Gas

Gas reflects ultrasound and obscures the tissues behind it through refraction and shadowing. Intestinal gas can obscure the liver, pancreas, para-aortic lymph nodes, uterus and ovaries. Sometimes it is easy to move the gas in the bowel: for example, if the urinary bladder is full, the uterus and the ovaries are nearly always easily seen because the bowel is pushed upwards out of the field of view. In other cases, oblique, lateral, or posterior scans with the patient sitting or standing may be necessary (Fig. 19).

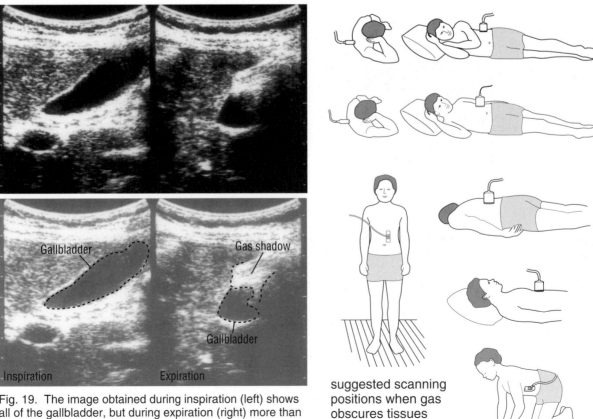

suggested scanning positions when gas obscures tissues

Fig. 19. The image obtained during inspiration (left) shows all of the gallbladder, but during expiration (right) more than half the gallbladder is obscured by bowel gas.

Reverberation

Reverberation occurs when the ultrasound beam passes from one tissue to another with a very different acoustic impedance, e.g. from intestinal gas to liver or ribs: the reverberation can obscure tissues that lie behind the gas (Fig. 20a).

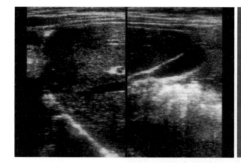
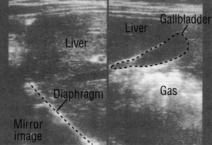

Fig. 20a. Gas artefacts. Left: there are repeated images of the liver behind the diaphragm; these are artefactual, caused by air in the lungs. Right: characteristic intestinal gas artefacts below the gallbladder might be interpreted as body structures.

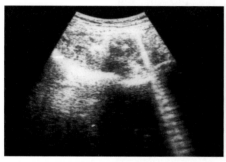
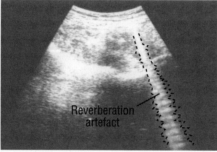

Fig. 20b. Reverberations: the lines are caused by multiple reflections of the gas between the bubble and the body surface. Gas artefacts can obscure underlying structures by absorption, oblique reflection and refraction.

Reverberations can completely change the image, producing either parallel lines or a mirror image. For example, reverberations between parallel layers of tissue below the skin may be seen as parallel lines in the urinary bladder (Fig. 20c).

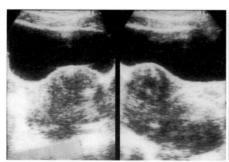
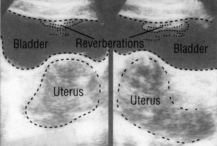

Fig. 20c. When the uterus is scanned through a full urinary bladder, the parallel layers in the abdominal wall may cause reverberation, seen as anterior echoes in the otherwise echo-free bladder. The transverse scan (left) looks different from the longitudinal scan (right) because of the different position of the transducer.

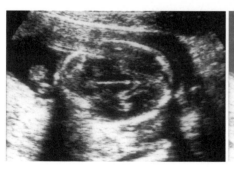
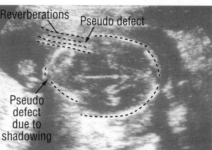

Fig. 20d. Shadowing and reverberation of ultrasound waves in the subcutaneous layers of this fetal head give false impressions of defects in the skull.

Incomplete imaging

Artefacts due to incomplete imaging are a source of error, since only that part of the tissue or any object that is actually in the acoustic beam will be imaged. Thus, in pregnancy, only part of a fetal bone may appear on the image because the remainder is not within the beam. As a result, the bone may appear to be incomplete or shorter than it really is (Fig. 21a, b).

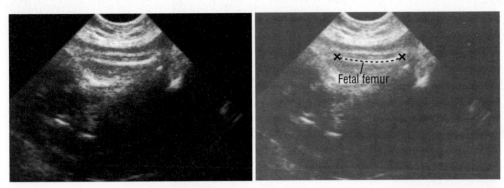

Fig. 21a. An incompletely imaged bone.

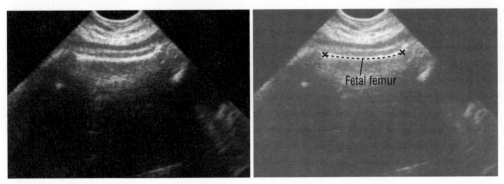

Fig. 21b. The same bone now fully imaged.

In practice, the most important artefact of this type occurs when needle biopsy or aspiration is guided by ultrasound. Whenever the tip of the needle is not within the scanning plane, it will not be seen on the screen, and the image will give the impression of a much shorter needle (Fig. 21c) (see also Chapter 22, p.317).

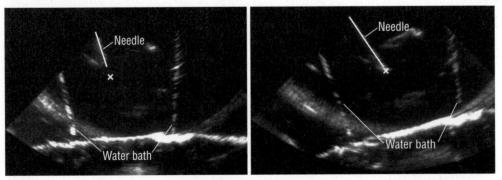

Fig. 21c. Images of a needle in a water bath. On the left, the needle is not entirely in the scanning plane and therefore appears shorter than it really is (the cross indicates the actual depth). On the right, the whole needle is imaged.

An ultrasound examination is a search.

Every ultrasound examination should provide three-dimensional information about the area under investigation *and* all the neighbouring organs. This will require multiple scans in different projections. Very seldom will a single scan in one plane provide enough information to allow the correct diagnosis to be made. Do not hesitate to make multiple scans.

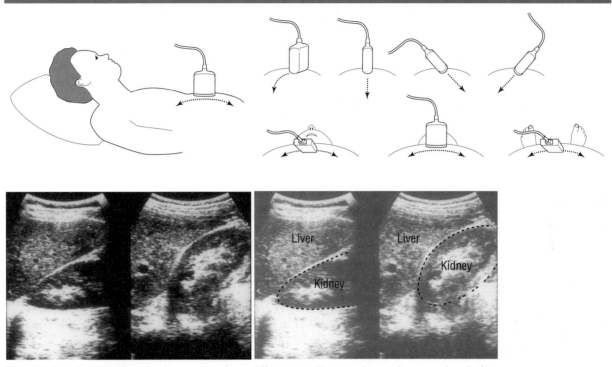

Fig. 22. Imaging the same body structure from different positions and transducer angles. Left: only the upper pole of the kidney is well seen. Right: the upper pole is blurred, but the rest of the kidney is seen clearly.

If you cannot see what is needed, turn the patient over on each side: or turn the patient half over (oblique); or examine while the patient is standing or on hands and knees.

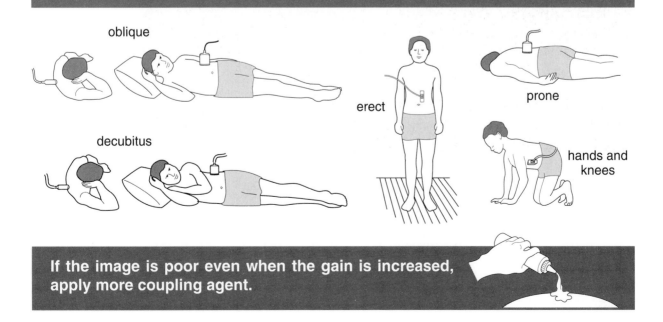

oblique

decubitus

erect

prone

hands and knees

If the image is poor even when the gain is increased, apply more coupling agent.

Quality control

Every ultrasound unit should be checked every day before clinical use. Although some basic quality control is essential, thorough and reliable quality control requires complex electronic and physical instrumentation. Only a trained physicist can do this properly and it is not usually practical outside a major department. However, simple quality control is not difficult and should be done regularly.

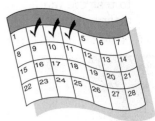

Ultrasound grey scale commercial "phantoms" allow regular checking of the resolution and sensitivity of the ultrasound unit and such checks should be made at least every three months and preferably more often.

Each machine must be checked, particularly when it is first delivered (see p. 22).

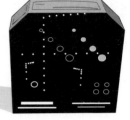

Ultrasound machines can vary in quality over a period of use.

Phantom

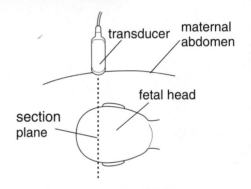

1. With good quality scans, it should be possible to demonstrate the cavum septi pellucidi in a 35-week-old fetus (Fig. 23) (see p. 247). When no phantom is available, this can be used as a clinical test to show that the scanner is working properly. The test should be carried out every three months.

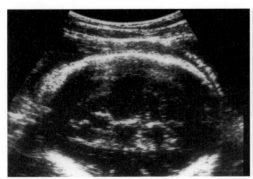
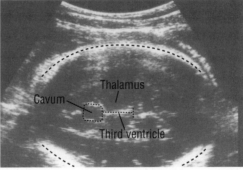

Fig. 23a. With any scanner, it should be possible to see the cavum septi pellucidi in the head of a 35-week fetus.

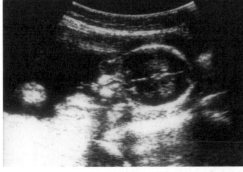
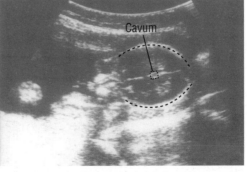

Fig. 23b. With a high quality scanner the cavum can be identified at a much earlier age.

2. The superior mesenteric artery should be visible as a round or oval hole close to the pancreas of a normal adult (Fig. 24). The easiest way to test the machine consistently is to image your own mesenteric artery. Keep a scan after each test for comparison.

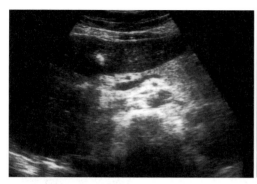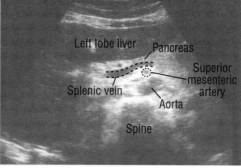

Fig. 24. Transverse scan: the superior mesenteric artery is shown as a round hole surrounded by echogenic fat, close to the pancreas.

3. Hepatic veins as small as 3 mm in diameter should be visible when scanned at 45° to the surface of a normal liver (Fig. 25).

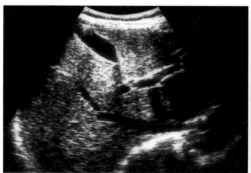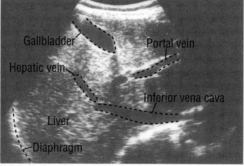

Fig. 25. A good quality scanner should demonstrate 3 mm veins in the liver. This should be used as one of the regular tests of image quality.

4. In a normal adult, the liver parenchyma should be slightly brighter than the nearby renal cortex (Fig. 26).

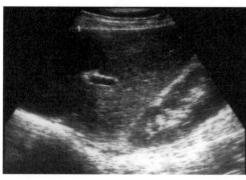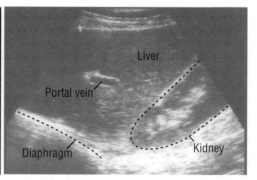

Fig. 26. Longitudinal scan through the liver and the right kidney: the normal liver parenchyma is more reflective than the normal kidney parenchyma. This is another useful way to check image quality.

Check the quality of your scanner at least every three months. Your patients deserve consistently accurate results. Keep records of all tests.

Notes

CHAPTER 4

Acoustic coupling agents

Introduction

If, during an ultrasound examination, air becomes trapped between the transducer and the skin of the patient, it will form a barrier that reflects almost all the ultrasound waves, preventing them from penetrating the patient. To obtain a good image, a fluid medium is needed to provide a link between the transducer and the surface of the patient. This fluid is called an acoustic coupling agent, often referred to as "gel".

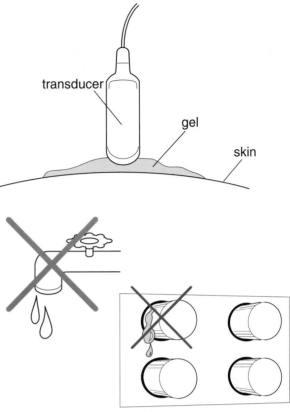

Water is not a good coupling agent because it evaporates rapidly owing to the heat of the body: it also runs away over the patient as the transducer is moved. It should only be used in an emergency, when nothing else is available.

Oil, either mineral or vegetable, is a good coupling agent, but when used for a long time may dissolve the rubber or plastic shielding of the equipment. If oil gets on the operator's fingers, as it inevitably will, it might damage the controls of the ultrasound unit.

The best acoustic coupling agent is a water-soluble gel. Many are commercially available, but they are usually expensive and sometimes difficult to obtain. It is not necessary to use a particular coupling agent with specified equipment, even though manufacturers often suggest that this is essential. Special coupling agents do not give a better image. The formula for a general purpose coupling agent for use with any transducer is given on p. 45.

The coupling agent is best applied using a squeeze bottle, from which it can be squirted onto the patient's skin. This avoids contamination. Any refillable plastic squeeze bottle is suitable, but it must be completely clean and dry before it is filled with the coupling agent. If there is an open wound, a skin rash or any other risk of infection, cover the transducer (or the skin) with thin plastic; put coupling agent on both sides of the plastic. The transducer must be cleaned after every patient.

The coupling agent should be removed with paper tissues, paper or cloth towels. It must be completely removed to avoid soiling the patient's clothing.

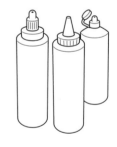

clean the skin

Remember: Whenever the image is not clear, or the sensitivity is reduced, *do not* adjust the controls until you have applied coupling agent to the patient's skin.

There can never be too much coupling agent.

Ingredients

Almost any hospital or commercial pharmacy should be able to prepare a suitable gel. All are based on synthetic resins, polymers of acrylic acid or other liquids that become water-soluble when neutralized with an appropriate alkalizing agent.

1. **Carbomer.** A synthetic high molecular weight polymer of acrylic acid cross-linked with allylsucrose and containing 56–68% of carboxylic acid groups. It is a white, fluffy, acidic, hygroscopic powder with a slight characteristic odour.

   Neutralized with alkali hydroxides or amines, it is very soluble in water, alcohol and glycerol.

   There are three carbomers: the most suitable is carbomer 940, which forms a clear gel in aqueous and non-aqueous vehicles. If carbomer 940 is not available, carbomer 934 or 941 can be used. However, they may not be quite so easy to mix (as described below) as carbomer 940.

2. **EDTA** (edetic acid). A white crystalline powder, very slightly soluble in water. Soluble in solutions of alkali hydroxides.

3. **Propylene glycol.** A colourless, odourless, viscous hygroscopic liquid with a slight sweet taste. Density = 1.035–1.037 g/ml.

4. **Trolamine** (triethanolamine). A mixture of bases containing not less than 80% of triethanolamine, with diethanolamine and small amounts of ethanolamine. A clear, colourless or slightly yellow, odourless, viscous hygroscopic liquid. Density = 1.12–1.13 g/ml.

Formula

The gel is prepared using these ingredients in the following amounts:

Carbomer	10.0 g
EDTA	0.25 g
Propylene glycol	75.0 g (72.4 ml)
Trolamine	12.5 g (11.2 ml)
Distilled water	up to 500 g (500 ml)

Preparation

1. Combine the EDTA with 400 g (400 ml) of water, making sure that it is dissolved, then add the propylene glycol.

2. Add the carbomer to the above solution and stir vigorously, if possible with a high speed stirrer, taking care to avoid the formation of indispersible lumps.

3. Wait until the mixture forms a gel and no more bubbles are observed.

4. Add the remaining water to make a total of 500 g of gel.

5. Stir carefully; *do not shake,* to prevent the formation of air bubbles in the gel.

The recommended formula is not known to irritate healthy skin or stain clothing, and is easy to clean off.

This gel may become more liquid when the patient is sweating, because it is affected by a high concentration of salts. This can be avoided by cleaning and drying the skin before applying the gel. If left in direct sunlight, the gel may liquefy. It is incompatible with bivalent or trivalent cations, such as calcium, magnesium and aluminium; if prolonged storage is likely, it is wise to store the gel in the dark. The stability of carbomer is considerably influenced by the pH, which must be maintained between 5 and 10. Outside these limits, the viscosity will fall.

CHAPTER 5

Abdomen

Indications

When the clinical symptoms indicate a particular organ, refer to the appropriate section, e.g. liver, spleen, aorta, pancreas, kidney, etc.

Indications for general abdominal scans:

1. Localized abdominal pain with indefinite clinical features.
2. Suspected intra-abdominal abscess. Pyrexia of unknown origin.
3. Nonspecific abdominal mass.
4. Suspected intra-abdominal fluid (ascites).
5. Abdominal trauma.

Preparation

1. **Preparation of the patient**. The patient should take *nothing* by mouth for 8 hours preceding the examination. If fluid is essential to prevent dehydration, only water should be given. If the symptoms are acute, proceed with the examination. Infants—clinical condition permitting—should be given *nothing* by mouth for 3 hours preceding the examination.

   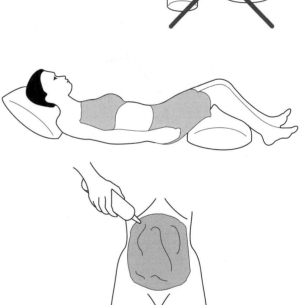

   As the examination progresses, and if there is no clinical contraindication, it may be helpful to give the patient water to drink, especially when scanning the pancreas, the lower abdomen and pelvis (see p. 113 and p. 196).

2. **Position of the patient**. The patient should lie comfortably on his/her back (supine). The head may rest on a small pillow and, if there is much abdominal tenderness, a pillow may also be placed under the patient's knees.

   Cover the abdomen with coupling agent.

   The patient can be allowed to breathe quietly, but when a specific organ is to be examined, the patient should hold the breath *in*.

3. **Choice of transducer**. Use a 3.5 MHz transducer for adults. Use a 5 MHz transducer for children or for thin adults. Curvilinear or sector transducers are preferable when available.

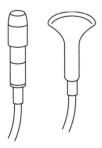
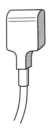

3.5 MHz
adults

5 MHz
children

4. **Setting the correct gain.** Start by placing the transducer centrally at the top of the abdomen (the xiphoid angle) and ask the patient to take a deep breath and hold it *in*.

Angle the transducer beam towards the right side of the patient to image the liver. Adjust the gain setting so that the image has normal homogeneity and texture. It should be possible to recognize the strongly reflecting lines of the diaphragm next to the posterior part of the liver (Fig. 27a).

The portal and hepatic veins should be visible as tubular structures with an echo-free lumen. The borders of the portal veins will have bright echoes, but the hepatic veins will not have such bright borders (Fig. 27b).

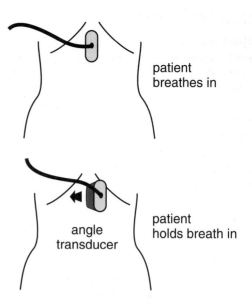

patient
breathes in

angle
transducer

patient
holds breath in

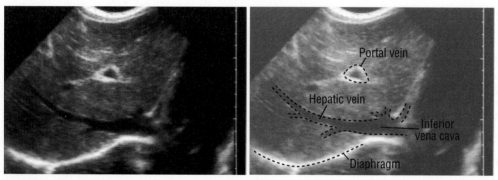

Fig. 27a. Longitudinal scan: the normal liver and diaphragm.

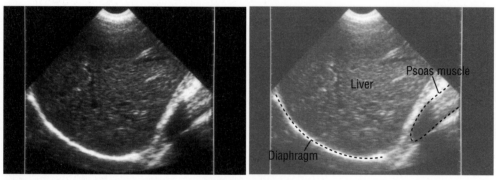

Fig. 27b. Longitudinal scan: hepatic and portal veins.

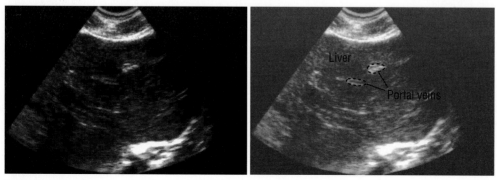

Fig. 27c. Transverse scan of a normal liver.

Scanning technique

After adjusting the gain, slowly move the transducer from the midline across the abdomen to the right, stopping to check the image approximately every 1 cm. Repeat at different levels. When the right side has been scanned, examine the left side in the same way. The transducer can be angled in different directions during this process to provide more information and better localization. It is important to scan the whole abdomen: if, after angling the beam, the upper parts of the liver or spleen are not seen, scanning between the ribs may be necessary.

After these transverse scans, turn the transducer 90° and start again centrally at the xiphoid angle below the ribs. Again, locate the liver and, if necessary, ask the patient to take a very deep breath to show it more clearly. Make sure that the gain settings are correct. When necessary, angle the transducer towards the patient's head (cephalad). Scan between the ribs to visualize better the liver and the spleen.

Below the ribs, keep the transducer in a vertical position, and move it downwards towards the feet (caudad). Repeat in different vertical planes to scan the whole abdomen.

If any part of the abdomen is not well seen with the transducer, the patient may be scanned while sitting or standing erect. If necessary, scan in the lateral decubitus position: this is particularly useful for imaging the kidney or spleen. Do not hesitate to turn the patient. Whenever there is any suspected abnormality, use the technique described in the appropriate section.

It is important to recognize:

1. Aorta and inferior vena cava.
2. Liver, portal vein, hepatic vein.
3. Biliary tract and gallbladder.
4. Spleen.
5. Pancreas.
6. Kidneys.
7. Diaphragm.
8. Urinary bladder (if filled).
9. Pelvic contents.

If any pathology is suspected during the abdominal scanning, refer to the appropriate section of this manual.

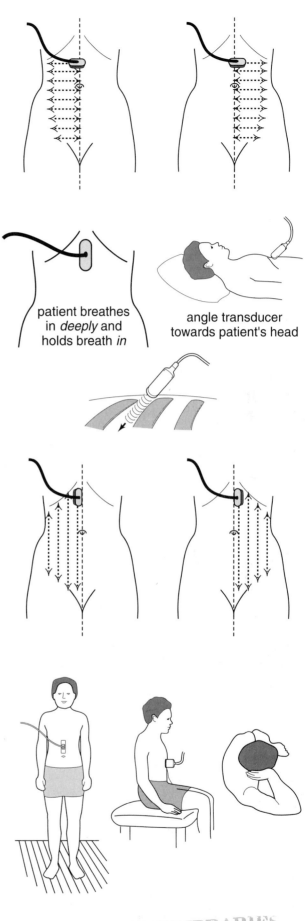

patient breathes in *deeply* and holds breath *in*

angle transducer towards patient's head

Notes

CHAPTER 6

Abdominal aorta

Indications

1. Pulsatile abdominal mass.
2. Pain in the midline of the abdomen.
3. Poor circulation in the legs.
4. Recent abdominal trauma.
5. Suspected idiopathic aortitis (patient under the age of 40 with vascular symptoms relevant to the aorta or major branches).

Preparation

1. **Preparation of the patient**. The patient should take *nothing* by mouth for 8 hours preceding the examination. If fluid is desirable, only water should be given. If the symptoms are acute, proceed with the examination. Infants—clinical condition permitting—should be given *nothing* by mouth for 3 hours preceding the examination.

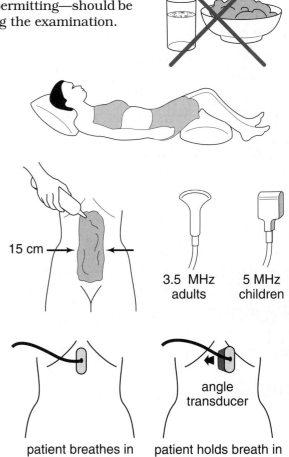

2. **Position of the patient**. The patient should lie comfortably on his/her back (supine). The head may rest on a small pillow and, if there is much abdominal tenderness, a pillow may also be placed under the patient's knees.

   Apply coupling agent down the midline of the abdomen over a width of 15 cm from below the ribs to the pubic symphysis.

   Scanning is best performed with the patient holding the breath in, but he/she may breathe quietly until a specific region needs more careful examination.

   15 cm

   3.5 MHz adults   5 MHz children

3. **Choice of transducer**. Use a 3.5 MHz transducer for adults. Use a 5 MHz transducer for children or thin adults.

4. **Setting the correct gain**. Start by placing the transducer centrally at the top of the abdomen (the xiphoid angle).

   Angle the beam to the right side of the patient to image the liver; adjust the gain to obtain the best image (see p. 50).

   angle transducer

   patient breathes in   patient holds breath in

Scanning technique

Move the transducer back to the midline and move it slowly towards the left until a pulsatile tubular structure is located. Follow this downwards to below the umbilicus, where the structure can be seen to divide: this is the bifurcation of the aorta (Fig. 28a, b).

Use transverse imaging to measure the cross-sectional diameter of the aorta at various levels. Image the iliac arteries by angling slightly to the right or left just below the bifurcation of the aorta.

umbilicus

aorta   transducer

iliac

Whenever a localized irregularity or variation is seen in the aorta (Fig. 28c), scan transversely at that level and closely above and below it. In elderly patients, the course of the aorta may vary and there can be some displacement or change in direction, but the diameter of the aorta should not change significantly. If the aorta cannot be identified, scan through the back towards the left kidney.

Gas

If there is intervening bowel gas, apply gentle pressure and angle the transducer; use an oblique or lateral projection if necessary, and scan from either side of the spine. Occasionally an erect scan may be used to displace gas-filled bowel.

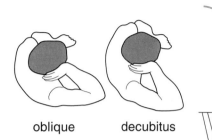

oblique   decubitus

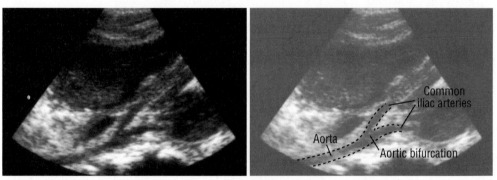

Fig. 28a. Longitudinal scan: a normal aorta.

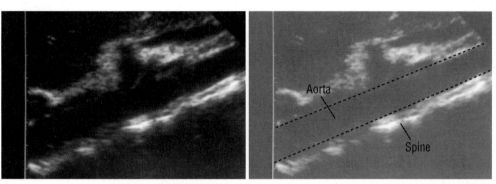

Fig. 28b. Coronal scan: the lower aorta, aortic bifurcation.

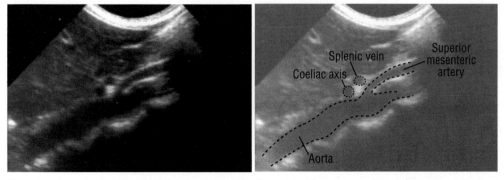

Fig. 28c. Longitudinal scan: the irregular aorta of an elderly patient.

When the aorta is being scanned, the coeliac artery and the superior mesenteric artery are important landmarks.

Normal abdominal aorta

The normal cross-sectional diameter of the adult aorta, measured as the maximum internal diameter, varies from about 3 cm at the xiphoid to about 1 cm at the bifurcation. Transverse and vertical diameters should be the same.

Measurements should be taken at various points down the length of the aorta. Any significant increase in diameter caudally (towards the feet) is abnormal (Fig. 29).

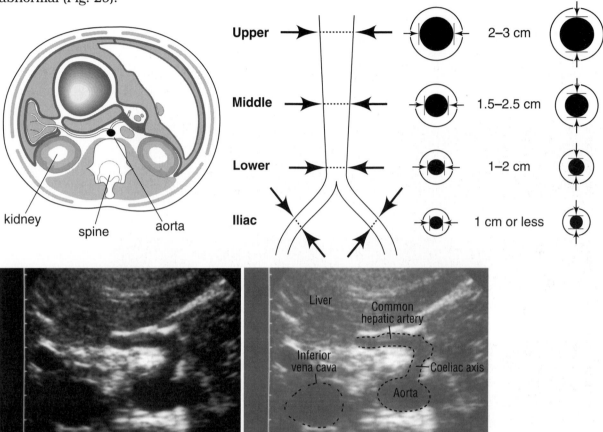

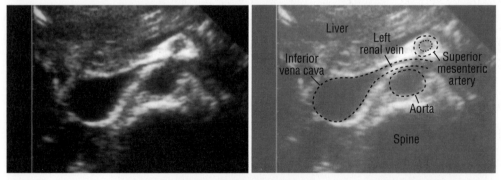

Fig. 29a. Transverse scan: the upper abdominal aorta and the coeliac axis.

Fig. 29b. Transverse scan: the mid-abdominal aorta and the superior mesenteric artery.

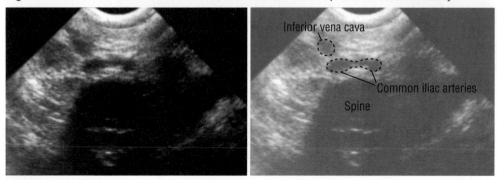

Fig. 29c. Transverse scan: the aorta at the level of the bifurcation.

Aortic displacement

The aorta may be displaced by scoliosis, a retroperitoneal mass or by para-aortic lymph nodes; in some patients these can mimic an aneurysm. Careful transverse scans will be needed to identify the pulsating aorta: lymph nodes or other extra-aortic masses will be seen posteriorly or surrounding the aorta (Fig. 30).

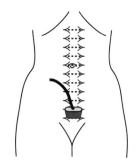

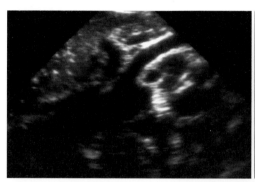
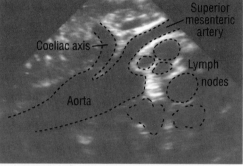

Fig. 30a. Longitudinal scan: the abdominal aorta is displaced by enlarged lymph nodes.

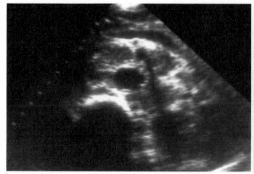
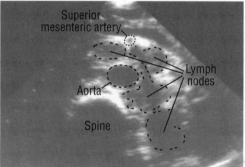

Fig. 30b. Transverse scan: the abdominal aorta is almost surrounded by enlarged lymph nodes.

If any cross-section of the aorta is more than 5 cm in diameter, urgent referral for clinical assessment is required. There is a high risk that an aorta of this size will rupture.

Aneurysm

A significant increase in the diameter of the aorta as it descends caudally (towards the pelvis) is abnormal; also, any section of the aorta that has a diameter greater than normal is likely to be aneurysmally dilated. However, aneurysm must be distinguished from dissection (p. 60), and, in elderly patients, marked tortuosity may be misleading. An aneurysm may be focal or diffuse, symmetrical or asymmetrical (Fig. 31a, b). Internal reflections may be due to a clot (thrombus) which may cause local narrowing of the lumen (Fig. 31c). When there is a thrombus, measurements must include both the thrombus and the echo-free lumen. It is also important to measure the length of the abnormal section (see also Aortic dissection, p. 60, and Idiopathic aortitis, p. 63).

A "horseshoe kidney" or a mass, e.g. lymph nodes, may also be mistaken clinically for a pulsating aneurysm. A horseshoe kidney will be anechoic and will appear to pulsate because it lies across the aorta. Transverse and, if necessary, angled scans should distinguish the aorta from the renal tissue.

> **The cross-section of the aorta should not exceed 3 cm at any level. If the diameter is more than 5 cm, or if any aneurysm is increasing rapidly in size (a change in diameter of 1 cm per year is regarded as rapid), there is a significant probability of rupture.**

> **If a fluid collection is seen in the region of an aortic aneurysm and the patient complains of pain, the condition is serious. Leakage may have occurred.**

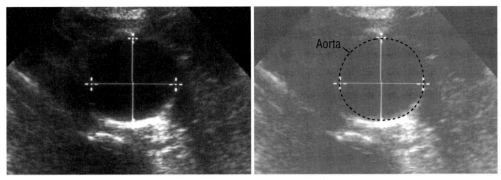

Fig. 31a. Transverse scan: a symmetrical aneurysm of the abdominal aorta.

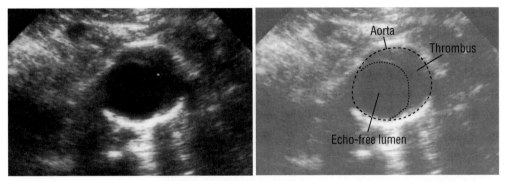

Fig. 31b. Transverse scan: an asymmetrical aneurysm of the abdominal aorta with thrombus in the lumen.

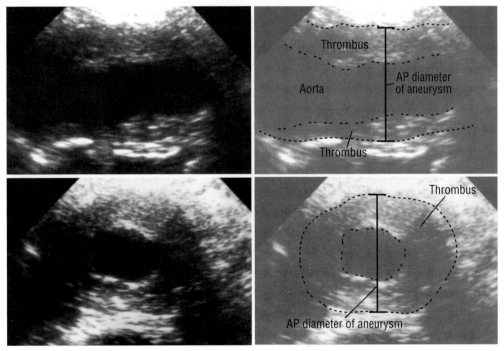

Fig. 31c. Longitudinal (upper) and transverse (lower) scans of an aortic aneurysm: the lumen is narrowed by a thrombus.

Aortic dissection

The aorta may dissect at any level (Fig. 32a) and over a short or long section. Dissection occurs most commonly in the thoracic aorta, which is difficult to image with ultrasound. The image of a dissection may suggest a double aorta or double lumen (Fig. 32b). The presence of intraluminal clot (thrombus) can also be very misleading because the lumen will then be narrowed (Fig. 31c, p. 59).

Whenever there is a change in aortic diameter, either enlargement or narrowing, dissection should be suspected. Longitudinal and transverse scans are essential to display the full length of the dissections; oblique scans are also necessary to show clearly the full extent.

When an aortic aneurysm or dissection is diagnosed, the renal arteries must be located prior to surgery to see whether they are involved (Fig. 32c). If possible, the state of the iliac arteries should also be demonstrated (see also pp. 56–59).

> **The clinical recognition of a highly pulsatile mass in the midline of the abdomen is an indication for an ultrasound scan.**

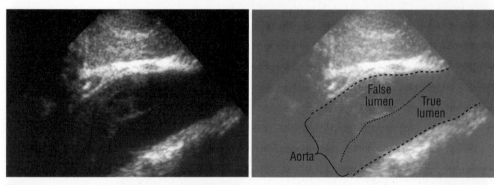

Fig. 32a. Longitudinal scan: an aortic dissection.

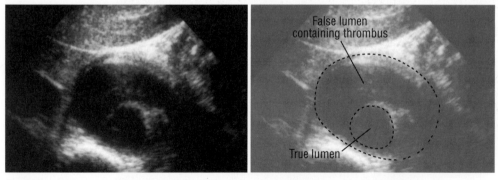

Fig. 32b. Transverse scan: the aorta appears to be double because of dissection.

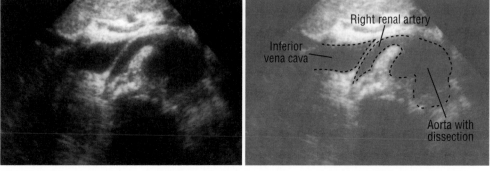

Fig. 32c. Transverse scan: dissection of the abdominal aorta at the level of the renal arteries.

Narrowing of the aorta

Any localized narrowing of the aorta is significant and should be visualized and measured in both diameters, with both longitudinal and transverse scans to show the extent of the narrowing.

Atheromatous calcification should be assessed throughout the length of the aorta. Whenever possible, the aorta should be traced past the bifurcation into the left and right iliac arteries, which should also be examined for narrowing or widening (Fig. 33a, b) (see p. 56 for normal measurements).

In elderly patients, the aorta may be tortuous or narrowed because of arteriosclerosis, which may be focal or diffuse. Calcification of the aortic wall will produce focal areas of acoustic shadowing on the scan. A thrombus may develop, especially at the bifurcation of the aorta, followed by occlusion of the vessel. Doppler ultrasound or aortography (contrast radiography) may be necessary. Each part of the aorta should be examined before stenosis or dilatation is diagnosed.

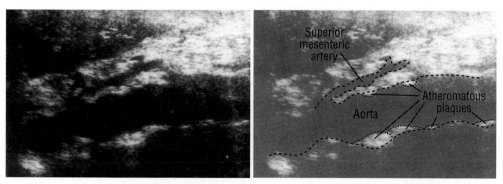

Fig. 33a. Longitudinal scan: stenosis of the abdominal aorta due to thrombosis close to a partially calcified atheromatous plaque.

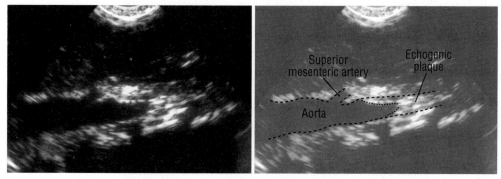

Fig. 33b. Longitudinal scan: the tortuous aorta of an elderly patient.

Aortic prosthesis

When the patient has had surgical repair of the aorta, it is important to assess the position and calibre of the prosthesis and, using transverse sections, to exclude dissections or leakage. Fluid adjacent to a recently inserted graft may be due to haemorrhage, but can also be due to localized post-surgical oedema or infection. Correlation with the clinical condition of the patient and follow-up ultrasound scans are essential. In all cases the full length of the prosthesis must be examined, together with the aorta above and below it (Fig. 34).

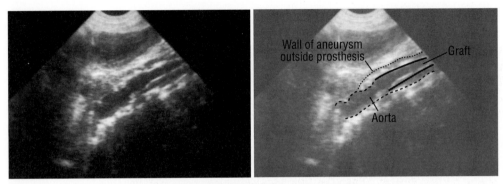

Fig. 34a. Longitudinal scan: an aorta with an intraluminal prosthesis.

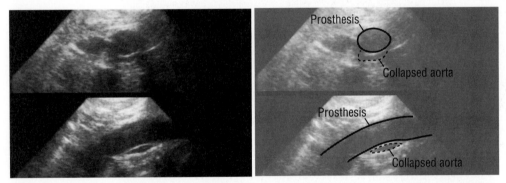

Fig. 34b. Transverse (upper) and longitudinal (lower) scans of an aneurysm of the aorta with a surgically placed prosthesis.

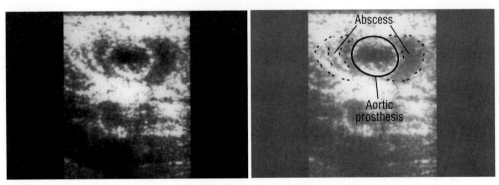

Fig. 34c. Transverse scan: an aorta with an infected prosthesis, which has resulted in an abscess. Blood leaking from an aneurysm would have the same appearance.

Idiopathic aortitis

The aneurysms of idiopathic aortitis occur most commonly in women under the age of 35 years but are sometimes seen in children. Aortitis may affect any part of the descending aorta and may cause tubular dilatation, asymmetrical dilatation or stenosis. Scanning in the renal area is essential to assess the patency of the renal arteries. In patients with aortitis, rescanning every six months is required, since an area of stenosis may subsequently dilate and become an aneurysm. Because ultrasound cannot image the thoracic aorta, aortography is needed to show the full extent of the aorta, from the aortic valve to the bifurcation and to demonstrate all the major aortic branches (Fig. 35).

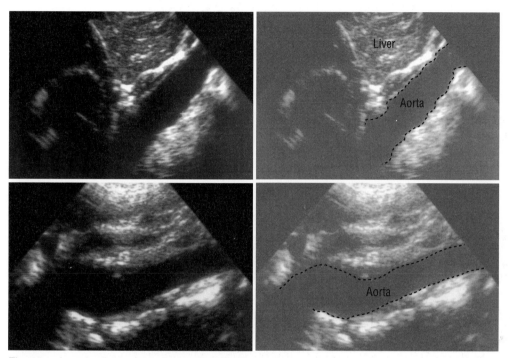

Fig. 35a. Longitudinal scans: Idiopathic aortitis in an 11-year-old girl. The upper abdominal aorta is dilated and irregular (upper), but becomes smoother and of normal diameter in the mid-abdominal region (lower).

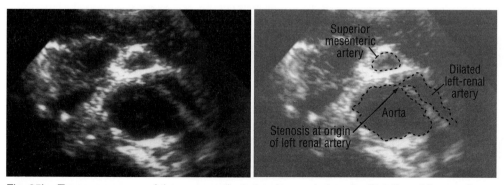

Fig. 35b. Transverse scan of the same patient showing post-stenotic dilatation of the renal artery.

64

Notes

CHAPTER 7

Inferior vena cava

Indications

1. Recent onset of dilated veins in the lower legs, with or without phlebitis (inflammation).

   Varicose veins are *not* an indication for caval ultrasound.

2. Multiple or suspected pulmonary emboli.

3. Renal tumour.

Preparation

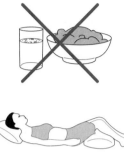

1. **Preparation of the patient**. The patient should take *nothing* by mouth for 8 hours preceding the examination. If fluid is essential to prevent dehydration, only water should be given. If the symptoms are acute, proceed with the examination.

2. **Position of the patient**. The patient should lie comfortably on his or her back (supine) with the head on a pillow. If necessary, a pillow may be placed under the knees.

   Apply coupling agent liberally down the midline of the abdomen over a width of 15 cm from below the ribs to the pubic symphysis.

3. **Choice of transducer**. For adults use a 3.5 MHz curvilinear transducer. Use a 5 MHz transducer for children or thin adults.

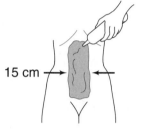

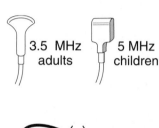

15 cm

3.5 MHz adults
5 MHz children

4. **Setting the correct gain**. Start by placing the transducer centrally at the top of the abdomen (the xiphoid angle).

   Angle the beam to the right side of the patient to image the liver; adjust the gain to obtain the best image (see p. 50).

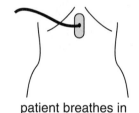

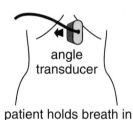

angle transducer

patient breathes in   patient holds breath in

Scanning technique

The patient is normally scanned while holding a deep breath in, or breathing gently. The breath should be held whenever any suspected abnormality is imaged.

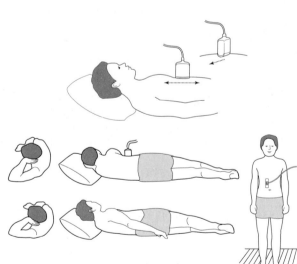

Scanning is normally longitudinal and transverse. If bowel gas prevents adequate imaging, oblique or lateral scans may be necessary to obtain a better image. Scanning with the patient erect may also be helpful.

Longitudinal scans will demonstrate the length and diameter of the inferior vena cava, which will be shown as a tubular, fluid-filled structure to the right of the aorta. Transverse scans will show the diameter at different levels.

Start by placing the transducer centrally at the top of the abdomen (the xiphoid angle). Angle the transducer to the right until the vena cava is seen along the right side of the spine.

When the patient takes a deep breath and holds it in, the vena cava will distend and be seen more clearly. Then re-examine the vena cava during active breathing: the wall of the vessel is thin, smooth and less dense than that of the neighbouring aorta. The vena cava appears in high contrast to the surrounding tissues.

Normal inferior vena cava

During respiration there should be change in the diameter of the vena cava, which normally collapses during inspiration and expands during expiration: this change allows recognition and differentiates the vena cava from the aorta. In transverse scans, the cross-section of the inferior vena cava is flattened or oval, whereas the aorta is round (Fig. 36a). The inferior vena cava will be flatter during inspiration and more oval during expiration, particularly forced expiration (the Valsalva manoeuvre) (Fig. 36b).

Once the vena cava has been recognized, careful scanning will usually show the hepatic and renal veins, and sometimes the iliac veins.

In elderly patients, the aorta may occasionally push the vena cava to the right or even lie in front it. Rarely, there may be two vena cava, one on either side of the aorta: these can be mistaken for hypoechogenic, enlarged lymph nodes. The variation in the size of each vena cava on respiration will help distinguish the veins from such solid tissues.

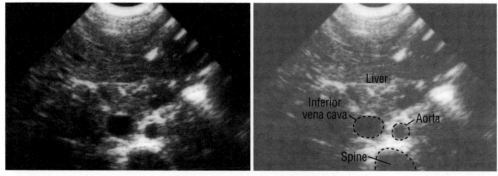

Fig. 36a. Transverse scan: the inferior vena cava and aorta.

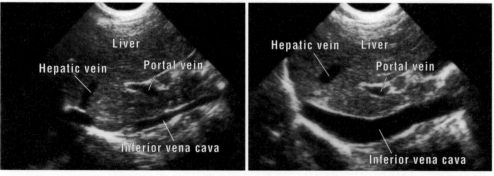

Fig. 36b. Longitudinal scans: there is flattening of the inferior vena cava during inspiration (left) compared with expiration (right).

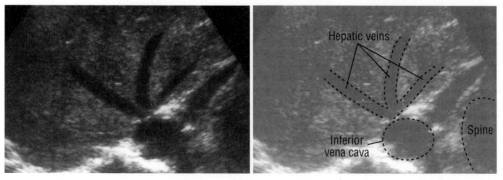

Fig. 36c. Transverse scan: the inferior vena cava and the hepatic veins.

Abnormal vena cava

Dilatation of the vena cava occurs when there is right-sided cardiac failure. There is no significant variation in diameter during respiration and the major caval branches may also dilate (Fig. 37a).

Compression of the inferior vena cava can be caused by hepatic tumours, enlarged lymph nodes or retroperitoneal fibrosis (Fig. 37b).

Anterior displacement of the vena cava can occur as a result of a spinal deformity, a spinal abscess (e.g. a tuberculous psoas abscess) (Fig. 37c) or a retroperitoneal tumour such as a lymphoma (Fig. 37d).

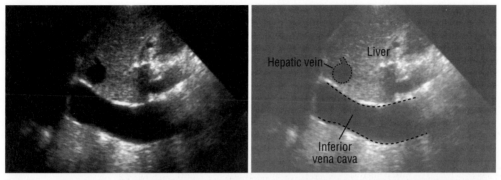

Fig. 37a. Longitudinal scan: dilated inferior vena cava in a patient in right-sided cardiac failure.

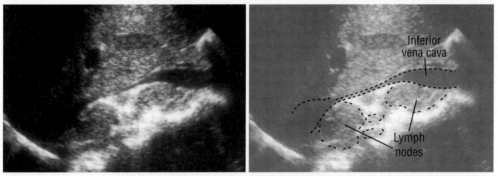

Fig. 37b. Longitudinal scan: compression of the inferior vena cava by enlarged lymph nodes.

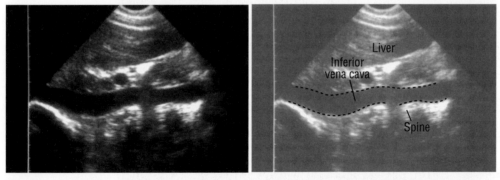

Fig. 37c. Longitudinal scan: anterior displacement of the inferior vena cava by the spine.

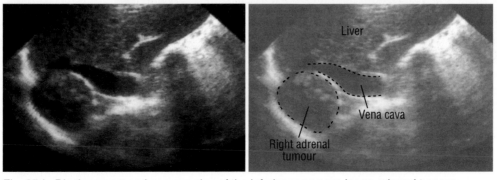

Fig. 37d. Displacement and compression of the inferior vena cava by an adrenal tumour.

Masses in the inferior vena cava

Well defined echogenic structures within the vena cava are probably due to thrombus or to an extension of a renal tumour (Fig. 38a); always check the outline of the kidneys when there are echogenic structures within the vena cava. A large venous channel parallel to the course of the vena cava may be a dilated ovarian or spermatic vein (Fig. 38b). If there are bright echogenic reflectors with acoustic shadowing within the vena cava, the clinical history should be checked to exclude an intraluminal filter (Fig. 38c).

Whenever thrombosis or tumour is suspected, it is important to examine the vena cava throughout its length to assess the extent of the lesion prior to surgery. Invasion of the vena cava occurs in renal cell carcinoma, hepatoma and adrenal carcinoma (see Chapter 13). If there is doubt, an inferior vena cavagram, computerized tomography (CT) or magnetic resonance imaging may be necessary.

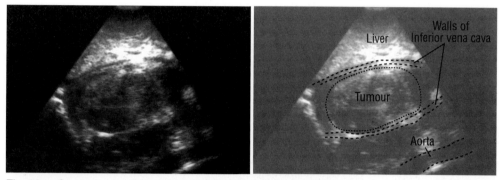

Fig. 38a. Coronal scan: tumour tissue filling the inferior vena cava.

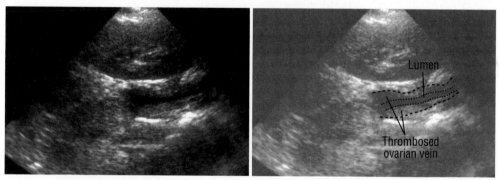

Fig. 38b. Coronal scan: thrombosis of the ovarian vein.

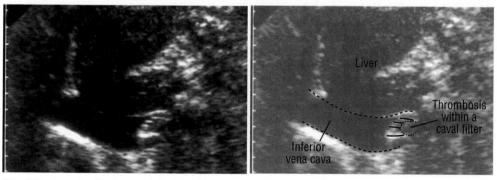

Fig. 38c. Longitudinal scan: inferior vena cava blocked by thrombosis in an intraluminal filter.

Notes

CHAPTER 8

Liver

Indications

1. Enlarged liver/hepatomegaly.
2. Suspected liver abscess.
3. Jaundice (see also pp. 107–109).
4. Abdominal trauma.
5. Ascites.
6. Suspected metastases in liver.
7. Suspected liver mass.
8. Right upper abdominal pain.
9. Screening for endemic echinococcosis.

Preparation

1. **Preparation of the patient**. The patient should take *nothing* by mouth for 8 hours preceding the examination. If fluid is essential to prevent dehydration, only water should be given. If the symptoms are acute, proceed with the examination. Infants—clinical condition permitting—should be given *nothing* by mouth for 3 hours preceding the examination.

   In many patients, additional information can be obtained from an antero-posterior supine radiograph of the abdomen. If there is acute pain, a radiograph should also be taken with the patient erect and must include the diaphragm to exclude subphrenic air from a perforated viscus.

2. **Position of the patient**. The patient lies supine.

   Apply coupling agent liberally, first over the right upper abdomen, then over the rest of the abdomen as the examination proceeds.

3. **Choice of transducer**. For adults use a 3.5 MHz transducer. For children or thin adults use a 5 MHz transducer.

4. **Setting the correct gain**. The gain setting should allow the diaphragm to be clearly seen; the liver (when normal) should appear homogeneous throughout its depth (Fig. 39). It should be possible to see clearly the normal tubular structures (the portal veins with bright edges and the hepatic veins without bright edges, see pp. 73 and 74). Hepatic arteries and bile ducts are not seen unless dilated.

   Before scanning a specific area, ask the patient to take a deep breath and hold it in.

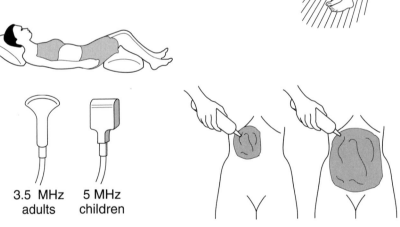

3 hours

supine   erect

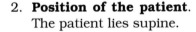

3.5 MHz   5 MHz
adults   children

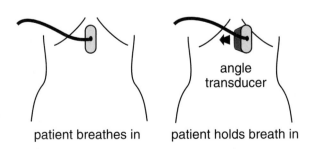

patient breathes in   patient holds breath in

angle transducer

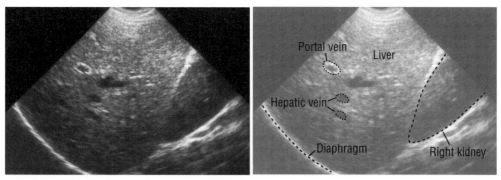

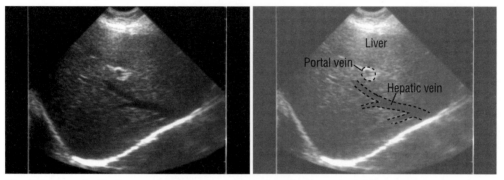

Fig. 39a. Longitudinal scan of a normal homogeneous liver.

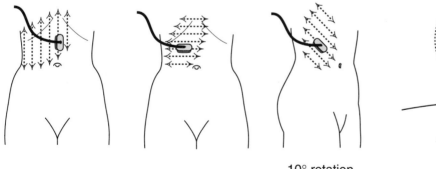

Fig. 39b. Longitudinal scan of the portal and hepatic veins in a normal liver.

Scanning technique

Scanning should be in sagittal, transverse and oblique planes, including scans through the intercostal and subcostal spaces.

Scanning should be done with a slow rocking movement of the transducer in all planes to obtain the best visualization of the whole liver.

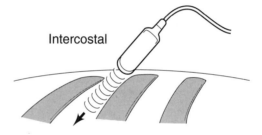

Intercostal

10° rotation, left side down

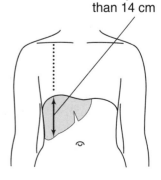

Usually less than 14 cm

It is difficult to measure accurately the overall size of the liver. In the mid-clavicular line, the longitudinal measurement from the diaphragm to the lower edge of the liver is usually less than 14 cm in an adult, but there is considerable variation.

Normal liver

The normal liver parenchyma appears homogeneous, interrupted by the portal vein and its branches which are seen as linear tubular structures with reflective walls. The thinner hepatic veins are non-reflective. In a normal liver, it should be possible to follow the hepatic veins to their confluence with the inferior vena cava. Hepatic veins can be made to dilate when the patient performs the Valsalva manoeuvre (forced expiration against a closed mouth and nose). The vena cava may be seen in the liver and may vary with respiration. The aorta may be identified as a pulsatile tubular structure behind and medial to the liver (Fig. 40).

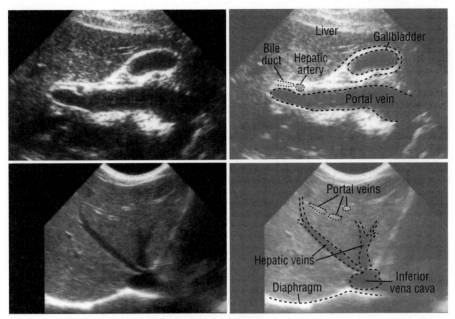

Fig. 40a. Oblique (upper) and transverse (lower) scans of the liver showing the portal and hepatic veins and the inferior vena cava.

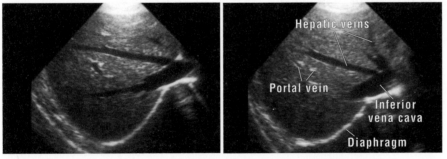

Fig 40b. Two longitudinal scans at slightly different angles showing the inferior vena cava, the hepatic veins and the bright (echogenic) walls of the portal veins.

The falciform ligament will be seen as a hyperechogenic structure just to the right of the midline in the transverse plane (Fig. 41a).

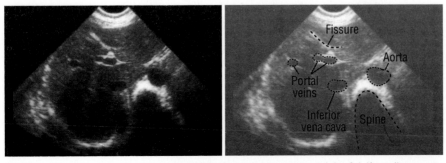

Fig. 41a. Transverse scan: the fissure of the ligamentum teres and the falciform ligament.

As well as the right and left lobes of the liver, it is also important to recognize the caudate lobe, limited posteriorly by the inferior vena cava and separated antero-superiorly from the left lobe of the liver by a highly reflective line. It is limited inferiorly by the proximal left portal vein. The caudate lobe must be identified because it may be mistaken for a mass (Fig. 41b).

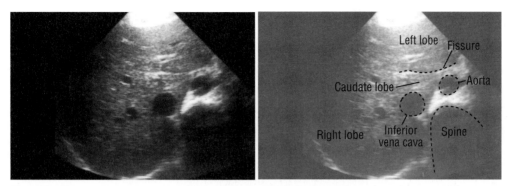

Fig. 41b. Transverse scan: the caudate lobe of the liver and the fissure of the ligamentum venosum.

The gallbladder and the right kidney must also be identified. The gallbladder will appear on a longitudinal scan as an echo-free, pear-shaped structure (Fig. 41c) (see also p. 94).

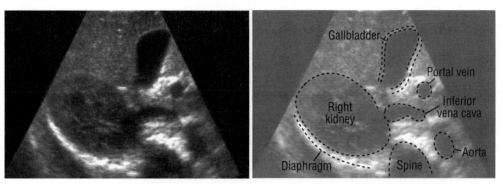

Fig. 41c. Transverse scan: the normal gallbladder.

The pancreas and vertebral column should be identified.

The echogenicity of the normal liver parenchyma lies midway between that of the pancreas (more echogenic) and the spleen (less echogenic) (Fig. 41d).

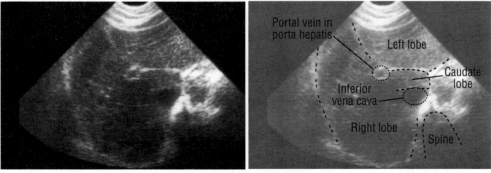

Fig. 41d. Normal echogenicity of different lobes of the liver.

Abnormal liver

Enlarged liver/hepatomegaly: homogeneous pattern

When the liver is enlarged but has a normal diffuse homogeneous echo pattern, consider the following:

1. **Congestive cardiac failure**. The hepatic veins will be dilated (Fig. 42a). The inferior vena cava does not vary on respiration. Look for a pleural effusion above the diaphragm.

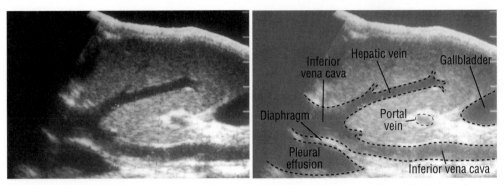

Fig. 42a. Longitudinal scan: hepatomegaly, dilated hepatic veins and a right-sided pleural effusion due to congestive cardiac failure.

2. **Acute hepatitis**. There are no characteristic sonographic changes, but the liver may be enlarged and tender. Ultrasound is useful to exclude other underlying disease and, when the patient is jaundiced, for differentiating between obstructive and non-obstructive jaundice (see also pp. 107 and 108). Ultrasound does not usually give further useful information on hepatitis (Fig. 42b).

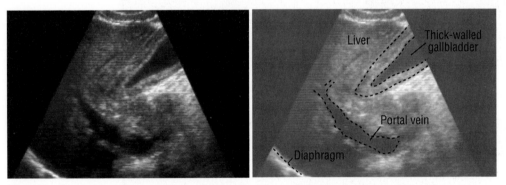

Fig. 42b. Transverse scan: oedema of the wall of the gallbladder, but normal hepatic parenchyma. The patient had acute hepatitis.

3. **Tropical hepatomegaly**. The only significant finding is liver enlargement, usually associated with splenomegaly.

4. **Schistosomiasis**. The liver can be either sonographically normal or enlarged, with thickening of the portal vein and the main branches, which become highly echogenic, especially around the porta hepatis. The splenic veins may be enlarged and, if there is portal hypertension, there is usually splenomegaly. An increase in collateral circulation may develop around the splenic hilus and along the medial edge of the liver. This is seen as tortuous, echo-free, vascular structures which must be distinguished from fluid-filled bowel. (Continued imaging will show peristalsis in bowel.) Periportal fibrosis may be due to either *Schistosoma mansoni* or *S. japonicum* (Fig. 43).

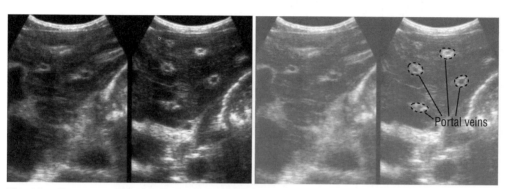

Fig. 43a. Transverse scans of left lobe of the liver, showing fibrosis around the portal veins (periportal fibrosis) due to *Schistosoma mansoni*.

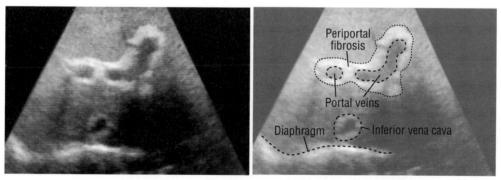

Fig. 43b. Transverse scan: periportal fibrosis due to *Schistosoma mansoni*.

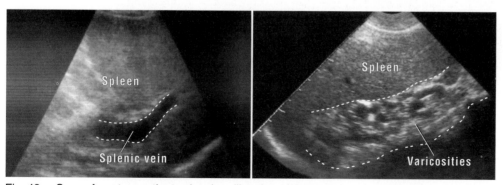

Fig. 43c. Scans from two patients showing dilatation of the splenic vein and multiple varicosities due to portal hypertension.

Enlarged liver: non-homogeneous pattern

1. **Without discrete masses**. When there is increased echogenicity in the liver parenchyma, with loss of the highly reflective edges of the peripheral portal veins, cirrhosis, chronic hepatitis or a fatty liver should be suspected. Liver biopsy may be required to establish the diagnosis. In severe cases, the region of the liver furthest away from the transducer may not be clearly imaged, so that the hepatic veins may not be identified (Fig. 44).

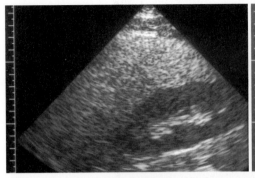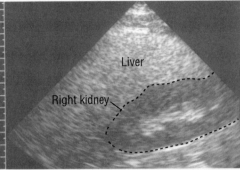

Fig. 44. Longitudinal scan: a fatty liver.

> **Cirrhosis is not excluded when an ultrasound scan of the liver appears normal.**

2. **With multiple echogenic masses**. Multiple masses of various sizes, shapes and echo textures, producing a non-homogeneous echo pattern throughout the liver, are consistent with:

- Macronodular cirrhosis. The liver is enlarged with echogenic masses of various sizes but with normal intervening tissue. The normal vascular anatomy is distorted (Fig. 45a). There is an increased risk of malignancy, but this can only be diagnosed by biopsy.

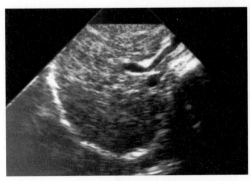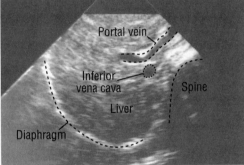

Fig. 45a. Macronodular cirrhosis.

- Multiple abscesses. These are usually ill defined, with strong back wall echoes and internal echoes (Fig. 45b) (see pp. 86–87).

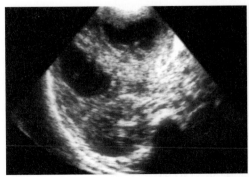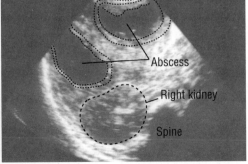

Fig. 45b. Transverse scan: multiple hepatic abscesses (amoebic).

- Multiple metastases. These may be hyperechogenic or hypo-echogenic and well circumscribed or ill defined, or both (Fig. 46). Metastases are often more numerous and more variable in size than abscesses; multinodular hepatocarcinoma can resemble metastases.

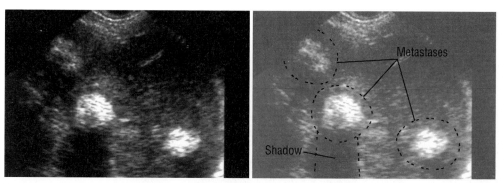

Fig. 46a. Transverse scan: multiple well-defined metastases in the liver.

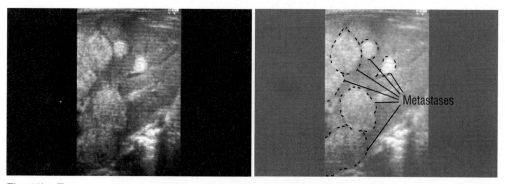

Fig. 46b. Transverse scan: multiple metastases in the liver, some well and others poorly defined.

- Lymphoma. This may be considered when there are multiple hypoechogenic masses in the liver, usually with irregular outlines and without associated acoustic enhancement. It is not possible to distinguish between lymphoma and metastases by ultrasound (Fig. 47).

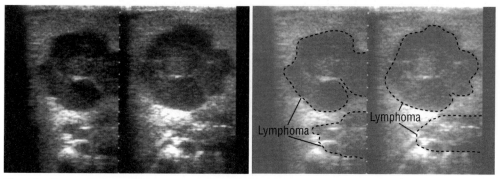

Fig. 47. Transverse scans: lymphomatous masses in the liver.

- Haematomas. These are often irregular in outline, with acoustic enhancement. However, when blood has clotted, the haematomas may be hyperechogenic. It is important to obtain a clinical history of either trauma or anticoagulant medication (see also p. 89).

The differential diagnosis between liver abscesses, metastases, lymphoma and haematomas is not easily made by ultrasound examination alone.

Small liver/shrunken liver

A diffusely increased echogenicity and distorted portal and hepatic veins in a shrunken liver are usually due to micronodular cirrhosis (Fig. 48). This is often associated with portal hypertension, splenomegaly, ascites, dilated splenic veins and multiple varices. The portal vein may be normal or small in the intrahepatic portion, but enlarged in the extrahepatic portion. If the lumen is filled with echoes, there may be thrombosis, which can extend into the splenic and mesenteric veins (Fig. 49). Some patients with this type of cirrhosis may have a liver that appears normal in the early stages.

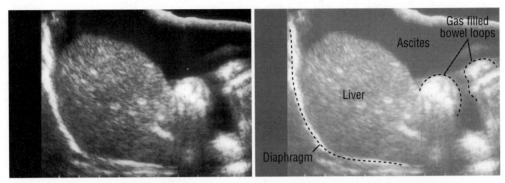

Fig. 48. Longitudinal scan: ascites and a small shrunken liver, the result of cirrhosis.

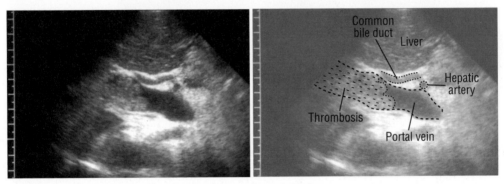

Fig. 49. Transverse scan: thrombosis of the main portal vein.

Cystic lesions in normal or large liver

1. **Well defined solitary cyst**. A well rounded, echo-free mass with acoustic enhancement, usually less than 3 cm in diameter, and often a chance finding without symptoms, is likely to be a solitary simple congenital cyst. A small hydatid cyst must also be excluded and cannot always be differentiated sonographically (Fig. 50a) (see pp. 82–83).

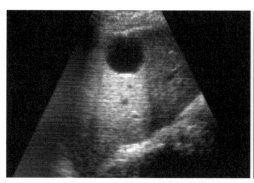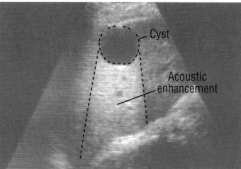

Fig. 50a. Transverse scan: a simple hepatic cyst with a sharp outline and acoustic enhancement.

2. **Solitary cyst with a rough irregular outline**. See liver abscess, p. 86.

3. **Multiple cystic lesions**. Multiple spherical cystic masses of varying sizes, completely echo-free with a sharp outline and posterior acoustic enhancement, may indicate congenital polycystic disease (Fig. 50b). Search for cysts in the kidney, pancreas and spleen; congenital cystic disease can be very difficult to differentiate from hydatid disease (see also p. 82).

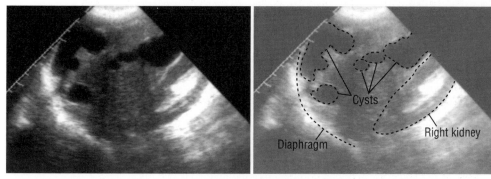

Fig. 50b. Longitudinal scan: congenital polycystic disease of the liver.

4. **Complex cyst**. Haemorrhage or infection of any cyst may result in internal echoes and resemble an abscess or necrotic tumour (Fig. 50c) (see pp. 85–86).

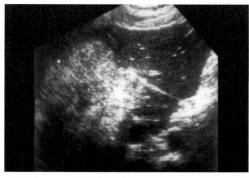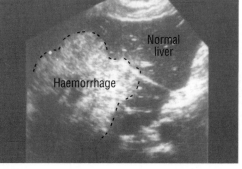

Fig. 50c. Haemorrhage into a cyst, which on ultrasound resembles an abscess or a necrotic tumour.

5. **Echinococcal cyst**. Hydatid disease can present a broad spectrum of sonographic features (Fig. 51).

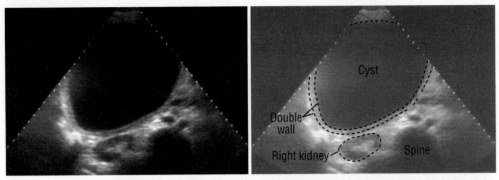

Fig. 51a. A simple, centrally echo-free intrahepatic cyst with a sharp outline and distal acoustic enhancement. Because of the host reaction, there is a double wall around this hydatid cyst.

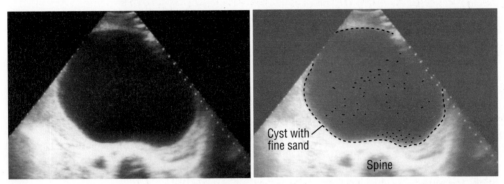

Fig. 51b. An echo-free mass containing fine internal debris due to hydatid sand. This may float freely or be at the bottom of the cyst.

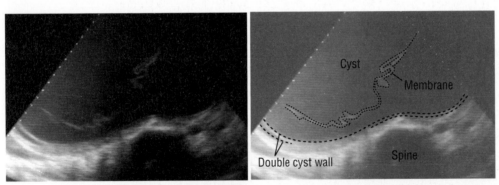

Fig. 51c. A well defined cystic mass with internal debris and a membrane floating within the cyst. This is pathognomonic of a hydatid cyst.

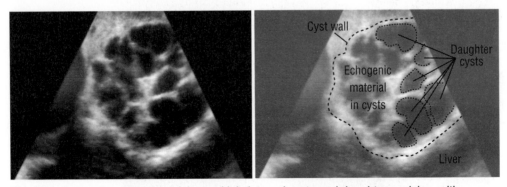

Fig. 51d. A complex mass containing multiple internal cysts and daughter vesicles, with echogenic material filling some of the cysts and the intervening spaces. This usually indicates a viable cyst.

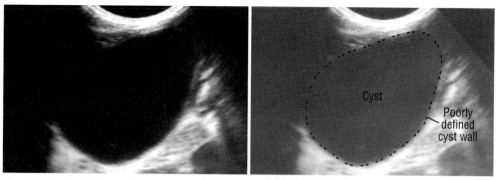

Fig. 51e. Infected hepatic cysts are difficult to differentiate from abscesses or other masses. The hazy outline of this cyst indicates the possibility of infection.

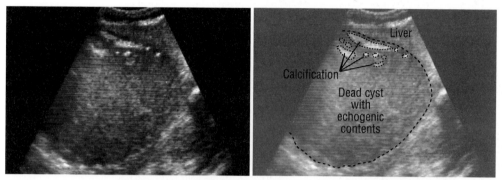

Fig. 51f. An echogenic mass with a sharp outline and calcification in the walls. This may indicate a dead hydatid cyst: hepatomas and liver abscesses seldom calcify (see pp. 85 and 86).

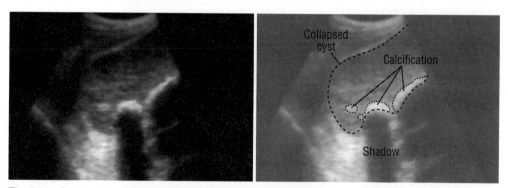

Fig. 51g. A hydatid cyst that has partially collapsed may resemble a scar.

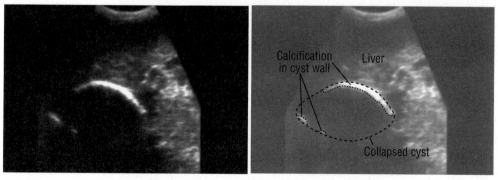

Fig. 51h. A small collapsed hydatid cyst with calcification in the cyst wall.

Before needle aspiration of an apparently solitary cyst, scan the whole abdomen and X-ray the chest. Hydatid cysts are usually multiple and may be dangerous to aspirate.

Differential diagnosis of liver masses

It may be difficult to distinguish hepatocellular carcinoma from multiple liver metastases or abscesses. Primary carcinoma usually develops as one large dominant mass, but there may be multiple masses of various sizes and patterns, which may have a hypoechogenic rim. The centre may become necrotic and appear quite cystic, with fluid-filled cavities and thick, irregular margins. It can be very difficult to distinguish such tumours from abscesses (Fig. 52) (see also p. 86).

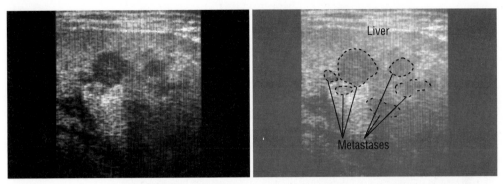

Fig. 52a. Hypoechogenic nodules with irregular outlines: metastases from colon carcinoma.

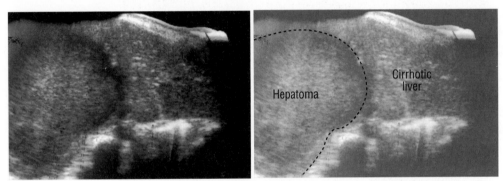

Fig. 52b. A large nodule in a cirrhotic liver. This is a hepatoma, but could be mistaken for an abscess.

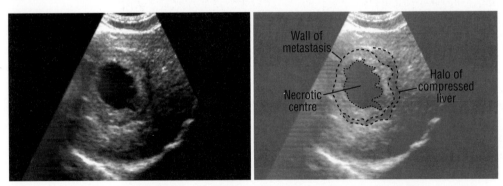

Fig. 52c. A mass in the liver with a surrounding halo and central necrosis: metastasis from breast carcinoma.

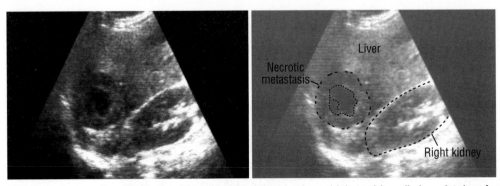

Fig. 52d. A necrotic metastasis with a central low-level echo, which could easily be mistaken for an abscess: clinical correlation is essential to make the correct diagnosis.

A single solid mass in the liver

Many different diseases may cause a solitary, solid mass in the liver. The differential diagnosis may be very difficult and may require biopsy (see also p. 84). A solitary, well defined hyperechogenic mass close to the liver capsule may be a haemangioma: 75% of haemangiomas have posterior acoustic enhancement without acoustic shadowing, but when large may lose hyperechogenicity and cannot be easily differentiated from a primary malignant liver tumour. Occasionally there will be multiple haemangiomas, but they do not usually produce clinical symptoms.

It can be very difficult to differentiate a haemangioma from a solitary metastasis, abscess, or hydatid cyst. A lack of clinical symptoms strongly suggests haemangioma. To confirm the diagnosis, either computerized tomography, angiography, magnetic resonance imaging or radionuclide scanning with labelled red blood cells will be necessary. The absence of other cysts helps to exclude hydatid disease. If there has been internal haemorrhage, the ultrasound images may resemble those of a necrotic abscess (Fig. 53a, b).

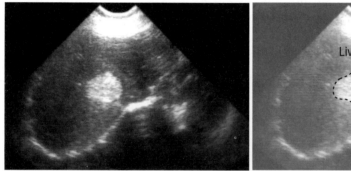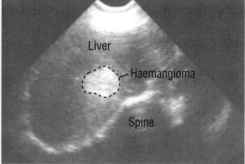

Fig. 53a. Transverse scan: haemangioma of the liver.

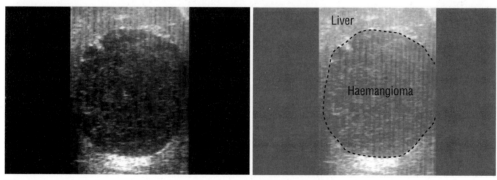

Fig. 53b. A large haemangioma of the liver, irregular in outline and hypoechogenic.

A single homogeneous mass with a low-level echo around the periphery is probably a hepatoma. However, hepatomas may also present with central necrosis or as a diffuse mass, can be multiple and may also infiltrate the portal or hepatic vein (Fig. 53c) (see pp. 81 and 84).

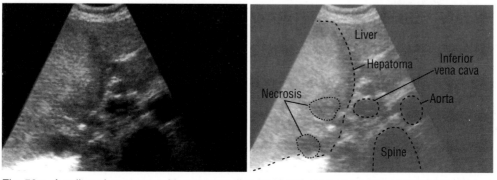

Fig. 53c. A solitary hepatoma with a surrounding low-level echo and areas of central necrosis.

Liver abscess

It is very difficult to differentiate between a bacterial abscess, an amoebic abscess and an infected cyst. All may be either multiple or single, and usually present as hypoechogenic masses with strong back walls, irregular outline and internal debris (Fig. 54a). There may be internal gas (Fig. 54b). Bacterial infection may also occur in an inactive amoebic abscess or in a healed amoebic abscess cavity. A necrotic tumour (see p. 84) or a haematoma (see p. 89) can also resemble an abscess (Fig. 54a, b).

Amoebic abscess

In the early stages an amoebic abscess may be echogenic, with poor edge definition, or even isodense and not visible. It will later appear as a mass with irregular walls and with acoustic enhancement. There is usually internal debris. As the infection progresses, the abscess may become well demarcated with a sharper outline: the debris may be finer (Fig. 54c). The same changes occur after successful treatment but the abscess cavity may remain for several years and be confused with a cystic mass. The scar of a healed amoebic abscess persists indefinitely and may eventually calcify (Fig. 54d).

Amoebic abscesses in the liver

- Usually solitary but may be multiple and of different sizes.
- More frequent in the right lobe of the liver.
- Usually near the diaphragm but can be anywhere.
- Respond to metronidazole or other appropriate treatment.
- May be isodense and invisible on the first scan. If suspected clinically, repeat the scan after 24 and 48 hours.
- Cannot be differentiated reliably from pyogenic abscesses.

Summary: amoebic and bacterial abscesses and hydatid cysts

	Number	Location	Internal wall	Contents	Clinical presentation	Response to metronidazole
Amoebic abscess	usually solitary; can be multiple	usually right lobe and peripheral	irregular	with debris	patient moderately unwell	yes
Bacterial abscess	multiple or solitary	usually deep	irregular	with debris	patient very ill	yes, if an anaerobic infection
Cyst	multiple or solitary	anywhere	sharp outline	anechogenic (other than hydatid)	patient usually asymptomatic	no

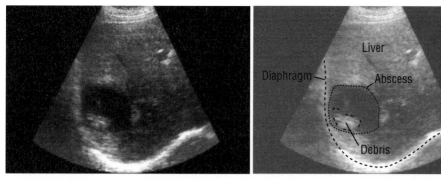

Fig. 54a. A pyogenic abscess in the liver.

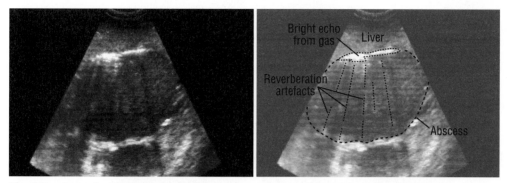

Fig. 54b. A gas-forming hepatic abscess with multiple bright reverberation artefacts.

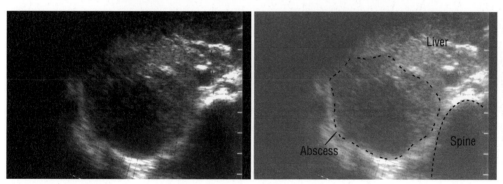

Fig. 54c. Transverse scan: an early amoebic abscess in the right lobe of the liver, hypoechogenic and irregular in outline.

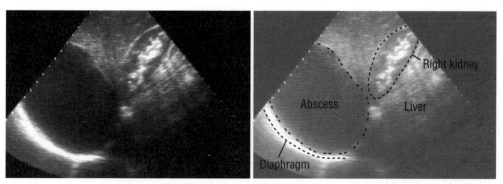

Fig. 54d. An amoebic abscess, which has been treated and now forms an almost echo-free subdiaphragmatic mass next to the right kidney. The walls are sharp and there is no acoustic enhancement.

Subphrenic and subhepatic abscesses

A predominantly echo-free, sharply delineated, crescentic area between the liver and the right hemidiaphragm may be due to a right-sided subphrenic abscess. Subphrenic abscesses are of various sizes and are often bilateral, so the left subphrenic region should also be scanned. If the abscess is chronic, the edges become irregular: septa may develop together with debris visible on ultrasound imaging (Fig. 55).

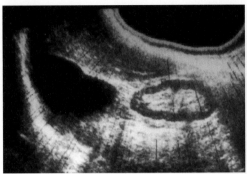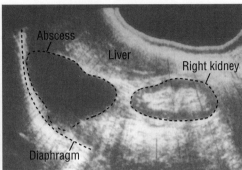

Fig. 55a. An acute right subphrenic abscess.

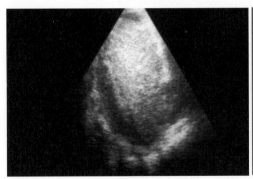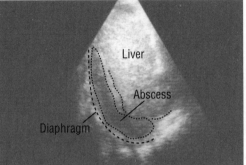

Fig. 55b. A chronic subphrenic abscess.

When using ultrasound to search for the cause of pyrexia of unknown origin, or postsurgical pyrexia, both left and right subphrenic regions should be examined.

The posterior aspect of the lower chest should also be scanned to exclude an associated pleural effusion (which can also be caused by pyogenic or amoebic liver abscess). A chest X-ray may be helpful. If a subphrenic abscess is found, it is necessary to scan the liver to exclude an associated amoebic or pyogenic abscess (Fig. 55c).

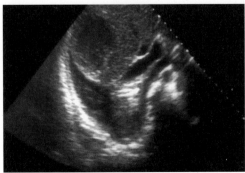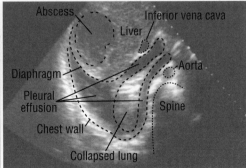

Fig. 55c. Transverse scan: a right pleural effusion and a pyogenic hepatic abscess.

Occasionally, a subphrenic abscess may extend to the subhepatic space, most commonly between the liver and the kidney, where it will show a similar echo pattern—either anechogenic or with complex echoes from internal debris.

Trauma to the liver

Haematomas

Ultrasound can reliably detect intrahepatic haematomas, which vary from hyperechogenic to hypoechogenic. However, the clinical history and symptoms may be needed to differentiate haematomas from abscesses (Fig. 56a) (see also pp. 86–87).

Subcapsular haematomas present as an echo-free or complex (due to blood clots) area located between the capsule of the liver and the underlying liver parenchyma. The outline of the liver is not usually altered (Fig. 56b).

Extracapsular haematomas present as an echo-free or complex (due to blood clots) area adjacent to the liver but lying outside the capsule. The ultrasound appearance may be similar to that of an extrahepatic abscess.

Any patient with an injury to the liver may have several haematomas, located within the parenchyma, below the capsule or outside the liver. Other organs, particularly the spleen and kidneys, should also be examined.

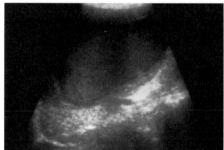
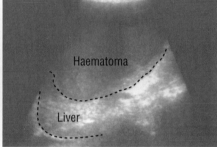

Fig. 56a. An intrahepatic haematoma.

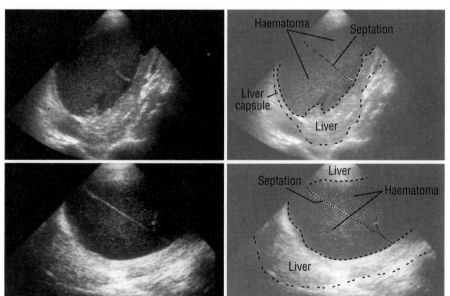

Fig. 56b. Two scans of a large subcapsular haematoma of the liver.

Bilomas

Fluid within or around the liver may be bile, resulting from trauma to the biliary tract. It is not possible to distinguish biloma from haematoma by ultrasound imaging.

Notes

CHAPTER 9
Gallbladder and biliary tract

Indications

1. Pain in the right upper abdomen: suspected gallstones and/or cholecystitis.
2. Jaundice.
3. Palpable right upper abdominal mass.
4. Recurrent symptoms of peptic ulcer.
5. Pyrexia of unknown origin.

Preparation

1. **Preparation of the patient**. The patient should take *nothing* by mouth for 8 hours preceding the examination. If fluid is desirable, only water should be given. If the symptoms are acute, proceed with the examination. Infants—clinical condition permitting—should be given *nothing* by mouth for 3 hours preceding the examination.

2. **Position of the patient**. Start with the patient lying supine: the patient may later need to be turned on to the left side or examined erect or on hands and knees.

   Apply coupling agent liberally to the right upper abdomen. Later cover the left upper abdomen also, because, whatever the symptoms, both sides of the upper abdomen should be scanned.

   Perform the scans with the patient holding the breath in or with the abdomen "pushed out" in full expiration.

3. **Choice of transducer**. For adults, use a 3.5 MHz transducer. Use a 5 MHz transducer for children and thin adults.

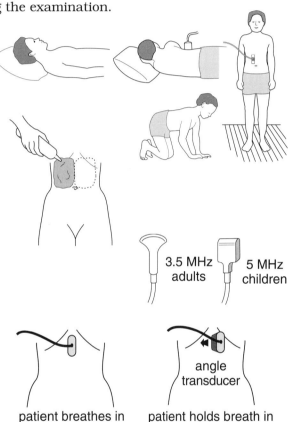

3.5 MHz adults · 5 MHz children

4. **Setting the correct gain**. Start by placing the transducer centrally at the top of the abdomen (the xiphoid angle). Angle the beam to the right side of the patient to image the liver; adjust the gain to obtain the best image (see p. 50).

angle transducer

patient breathes in · patient holds breath in

Scanning technique

Start with longitudinal scans, then transverse scans; add intercostal scans if needed. Then turn the patient on to the left side and make oblique scans at different angles.

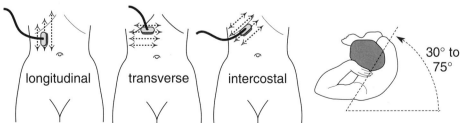

longitudinal · transverse · intercostal · 30° to 75°

If there is excessive gas in the bowel, examine the patient standing erect (sitting up will not usually displace bowel gas).

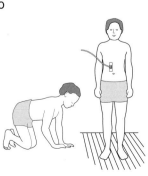

The hands/knees position can be used to demonstrate gallstones more clearly, allowing the stones to move anteriorly.

Normal anatomy of the gallbladder

On the longitudinal scan the gallbladder will appear as an echo-free, pear-shaped structure. It is very variable in position, size and shape, but the normal gallbladder is seldom more than 4 cm wide (Fig. 57).

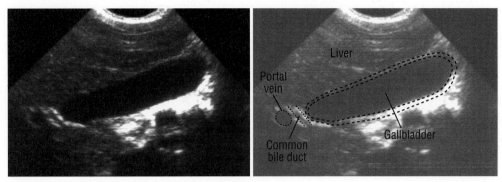

Fig. 57a. Longitudinal scan: normal full gallbladder.

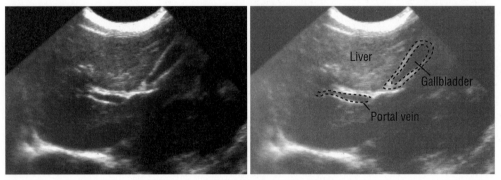

Fig. 57b. Longitudinal scan: normal, partially empty gallbladder.

The gallbladder may be mobile. It may be elongated and on scanning may be found below the level of the superior iliac crest (especially when the patient is erect). It may be to the left of the midline. If not located in the normal position, scan the whole abdomen, starting on the right side.

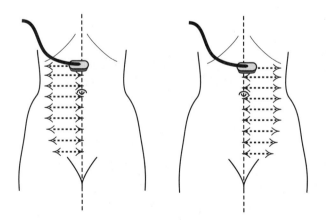

The thickness of the gallbladder wall can be measured on transverse scans; in a fasting patient it is normally 3 mm or less and 1 mm when the gallbladder is distended (Fig. 58) (see p. 104).

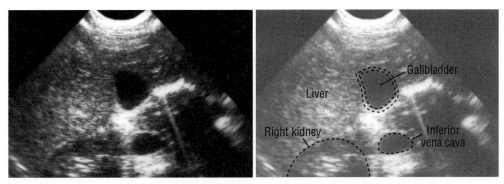

Fig. 58a. Transverse scan: normal, full gallbladder (wall thickness 1 mm).

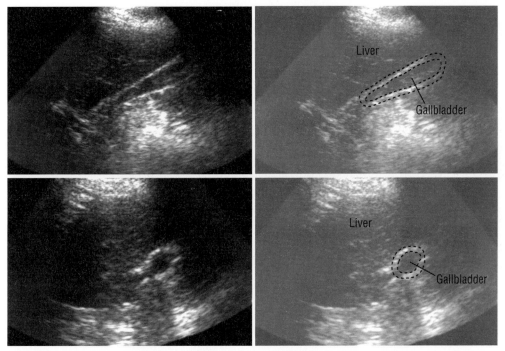

Fig 58b. Longitudinal (upper) and transverse (lower) scans of a contracted gallbladder (wall thickness less than 3 mm).

If the gallbladder is not identified in its usual position, scan the whole abdomen and the pelvis. If necessary, rescan after 6–8 hours, or ask a colleague to scan the patient.

Failure to demonstrate the gallbladder with ultrasound does not mean it is absent.

It is not always easy to identify the normal main right and left hepatic biliary ducts, but when visible they are within the liver and appear as thin-walled tubular structures. However, the common hepatic duct can usually be recognized just anterior and lateral to the crossing portal vein, and its cross-section at this level should not exceed 5 mm. The diameter of the common bile duct is variable but should not exceed 9 mm near its entrance into the pancreas (Fig. 59) (see also p. 108).

Scanning a jaundiced patient is discussed in detail on pp. 107–109.

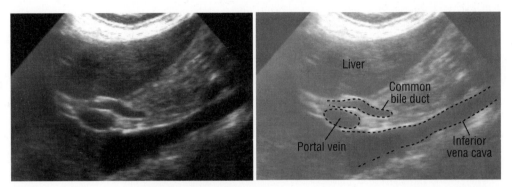

Fig. 59a. Oblique scan: normal common bile duct.

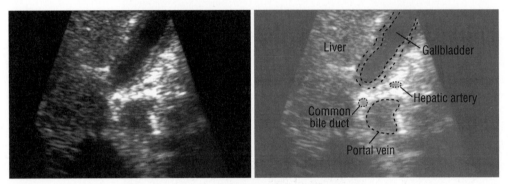

Fig. 59b. Transverse scan: the common bile duct at the porta hepatis.

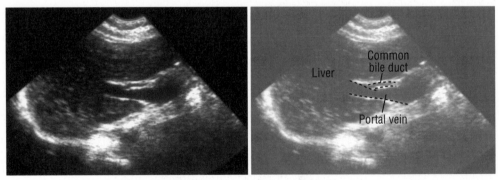

Fig. 59c. Oblique scan: the common bile duct at the porta hepatis.

Nonvisualization of the gallbladder

There are various reasons why the gallbladder may not be seen by ultrasound:

1. The patient has not been fasting: re-examine after an interval of at least 6 hours without food or drink.

2. The gallbladder lies in an unusual position.

   • Scan low down in the right abdomen, even as far as the pelvis.

   • Scan to the left of the midline and with the patient in the oblique position with the right side down.

   • Scan high under the costal margin.

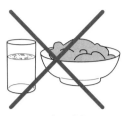

no food for
at least 6 hours

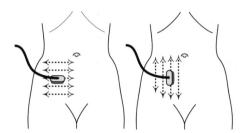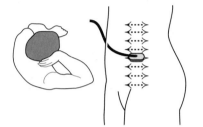

3. The gallbladder is congenitally hypoplastic or absent.

4. The gallbladder is shrunken and full of stones (calculi), with associated acoustic shadowing.

5. The gallbladder has been removed surgically: examine the abdomen for scars and ask the patient (or relatives).

6. The examiner is not properly trained or experienced: ask a colleague to examine the patient.

There are very few pathological conditions (other than congenital absence or surgical removal) that result in persistent nonvisualization of the gallbladder by ultrasound.

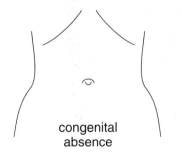

congenital
absence

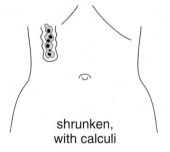

shrunken,
with calculi

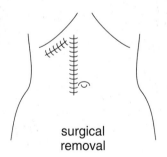

surgical
removal

No clinical judgement should be made if the gallbladder is not visualized, even after scanning in different positions.

Enlarged (distended) gallbladder

The gallbladder is enlarged if it exceeds 4 cm in width (transverse diameter).

The normal gallbladder may appear distended when the patient is dehydrated, has been on a low-fat diet or on intravenous nutrition, or has been immobilized for some time. If there is no clinical evidence of cholecystitis, and if the gallbladder wall does not appear thickened on ultrasound, give the patient a fatty meal and repeat the ultrasound examination in 45 minutes to 1 hour. A normal gallbladder will contract (Fig. 60a).

If there is no contraction, search for:

1. A gallstone or other cause of obstruction within the cystic duct. The hepatic and bile ducts will be normal. If there is no internal obstruction, there may be a mass or lymph node pressing externally on the duct.

2. A stone or other obstruction in the common bile duct. The common hepatic duct will be dilated (over 5 mm diameter). Examine the common bile duct for *Ascaris* (Fig. 60b): on a transverse scan, a tube within a tube is the "target" sign (Fig. 60c). Look for *Ascaris* also in the stomach or small bowel. Obstruction may be due to a carcinoma at the head of the pancreas (an echogenic mass), or where hydatid disease is endemic, cyst membranes in the common duct. (Scan the liver and the abdomen for cysts, and X-ray the chest.)

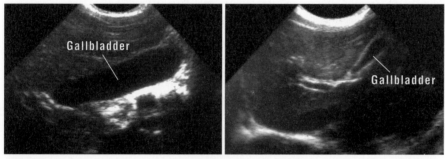

Fig. 60a. Left: the gallbladder is full. Right: the gallbladder has contracted after a fatty meal.

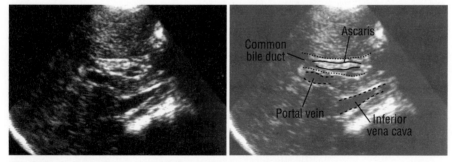

Fig. 60b. Longitudinal scan: *Ascaris* in the common bile duct.

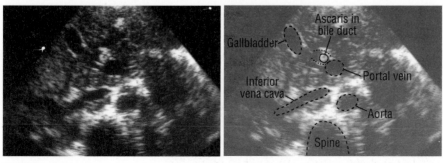

Fig. 60c. Transverse scan: *Ascaris* in the common bile duct: this shows the "target" sign.

3. If the gallbladder is distended with thickened walls (greater than 5 mm) and filled with fluid, there may be an empyema: local tenderness is likely. Check the patient clinically (Fig. 61).

4. If the gallbladder is distended with thin walls and filled with fluid, there may be a mucocele. This does not usually result in local tenderness.

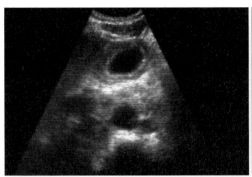
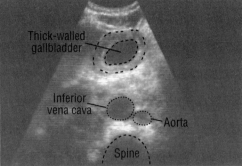

Fig. 61a. Transverse scan: a distended gallbladder with thick walls.

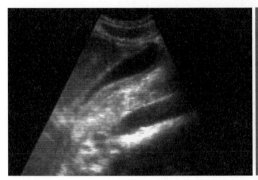
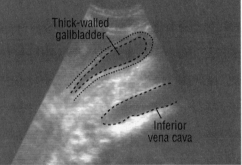

Fig. 61b. Longitudinal scan: the same distended, thick-walled gallbladder.

Acute cholecystitis

Clinically, acute cholecystitis is usually associated with pain in the right upper abdomen and with local tenderness when the transducer is (carefully) applied near the gallbladder. There may be one or more gallstones, probably including a stone in the gallbladder neck or in the cystic duct (see pp. 100–102). The walls of the gallbladder are likely to be thickened and oedematous, and, therefore, the gallbladder is not always distended. If the gallbladder has perforated, there is usually fluid adjacent to it.

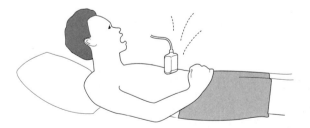

Gallstones do not always cause symptoms: exclude other disease even when there are gallstones.

Echoes within the gallbladder

Mobile internal echoes with shadowing

1. Gallstones can be recognized as bright intraluminal echogenic structures with an acoustic shadow. The stones may be single or multiple, large or small, calcified or non-calcified. The gallbladder walls may be normal or thickened (Fig. 62a, b).

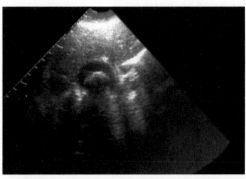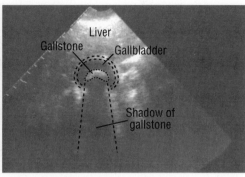

Fig. 62a. Transverse scan: a single stone in the gallbladder.

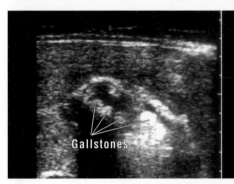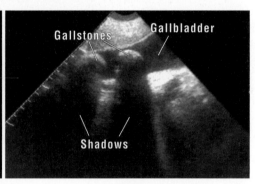

Fig. 62b. Longitudinal scans: multiple small gallstones (left); two large gallstones (right).

2. When gallstones are suspected but not seen clearly on routine scans, rescan with the patient oblique or erect. Most gallstones will change position within the gallbladder as the patient moves (Fig 62c, d) (see also p. 101).

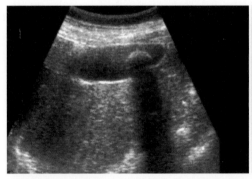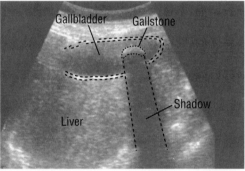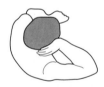

Fig. 62c. A gallbladder containing a large solitary stone.

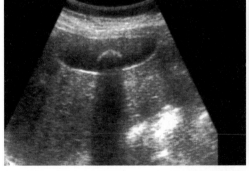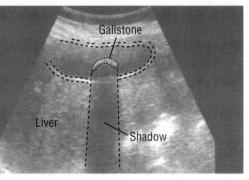

Fig. 62d. When the same patient is moved, the gallstone changes position.

3. If there is still any doubt, scan the patient in the hands/knees position. The gallstones will move anteriorly. This position may also be useful if there is excessive bowel gas (Fig. 62e, f).

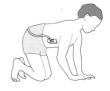

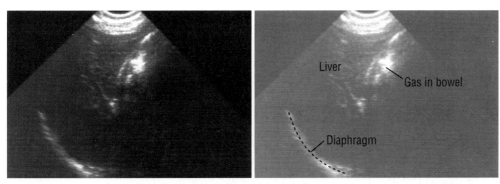

Fig. 62e. An unsuccessful scan, because the gallbladder is obscured by gas in the bowel.

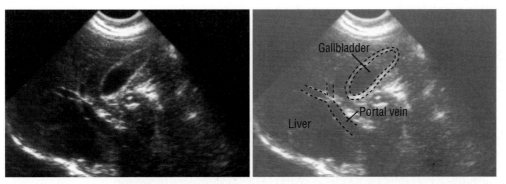

Fig. 62f. With the same patient in the hands/knees position, the gallbladder is seen clearly.

Ultrasound can reliably diagnose gallstones when they are in the gallbladder.

Ultrasound is *not* always reliable in recognizing stones in the bile ducts.

Gallstones do not always cause symptoms: exclude other disease even when there are gallstones.

Mobile internal echoes without shadowing

Scans should be taken in different positions. The common causes are:

1. Gallstones. Note that there will be no acoustic shadow if the stones are smaller than the diameter of the ultrasound beam (Fig. 63a).

2. Gallbladder sludge. This is thickened bile which produces fine dependent echoes that move slowly with a change in the position of the patient, unlike stones which tend to move quickly (Fig. 63b).

3. Pyogenic debris (Fig. 63c).

4. Blood clots.

5. Hydatid membranes. Scan the liver for cysts (see pp. 81–83).

6. *Ascaris* and other parasites. It is unusual for worms such as *Ascaris* to reach the gallbladder. They are more likely to be seen in the bile duct (see p. 98). In clonorchiasis the hepatic ducts will be dilated and irregular and there is often much intraductal debris (see p. 110).

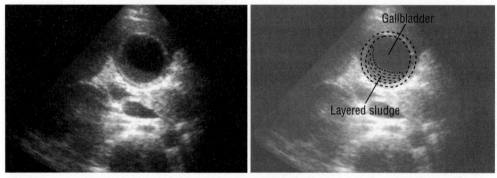

Fig. 63a. Transverse scan: the gallbladder is very distended and contains fine sludge. The distension was due to a small stone in the cystic duct, which did not produce an acoustic shadow.

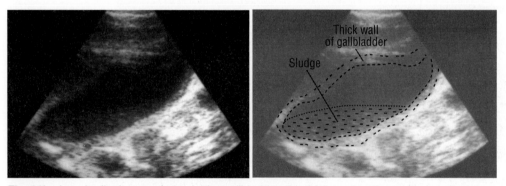

Fig. 63b. Longitudinal scan: sludge in the gallbladder: the thickened walls are the result of chronic inflammation.

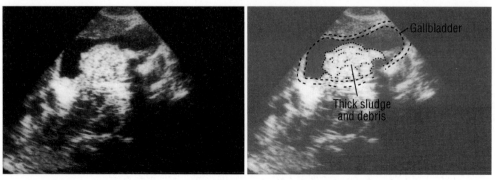

Fig. 63c. Thick sludge and debris in the gallbladder from pyogenic infection.

Nonmobile internal echoes with shadowing

The commonest cause is an impacted calculus (Fig. 64a): search for other calculi. The calcification may also be in the gallbladder wall: if the wall is also thickened, there may be acute or chronic cholecystitis, but it may be difficult to exclude an associated carcinoma (see p. 105).

Nonmobile internal echoes without shadowing

1. The most common cause is a polyp (Fig. 64b). It may be possible to identify the pedicle by using different scanning projections. There should be no acoustic shadowing, and changing the patient's position will not move the polyp but may alter its shape. Malignant disease may resemble a polyp but is more often associated with thickening of the gallbladder wall and does not usually have a pedicle. A malignant tumour is less likely to change its shape when the patient changes position (see p. 105).

2. A septum or fold within the gallbladder is not likely to be of any clinical significance (see p. 105).

3. A malignant tumour (Fig. 64c) (see p. 105).

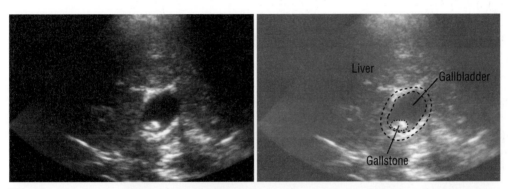

Fig. 64a. Transverse scan of the gallbladder: there will probably be distension when there is a stone impacted in the neck of the gallbladder.

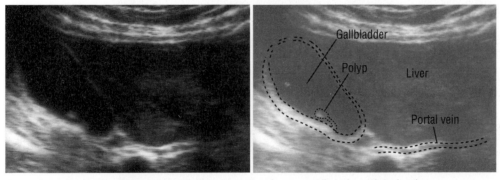

Fig. 64b. Longitudinal scan of the gallbladder showing a small pedunculated polyp.

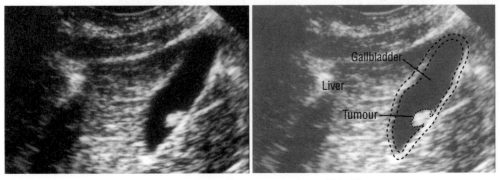

Figure 64c. Longitudinal scan: a small sessile tumour in the gallbladder.

Thick gallbladder walls

Generalized thickening

The thickness of the gallbladder wall is normally less than 3 mm and should not exceed 5 mm. When the thickness is between 3 mm and 5 mm, careful clinical correlation is needed. Generalized thickening of the gallbladder wall can occur in the following conditions:

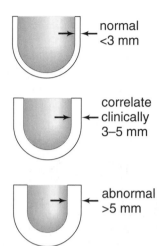

normal
<3 mm

correlate
clinically
3–5 mm

abnormal
>5 mm

1. Acute cholecystitis. This may be associated with an echo-free section in the wall or a localized fluid collection. Stones may be present: check the neck of the gallbladder (see p. 99).

2. Chronic cholecystitis (Fig. 65a). There may also be stones (see pp. 100–102).

3. Hypoalbuminaemia resulting from cirrhosis. Check for ascites, dilated portal veins and splenomegaly.

4. Congestive cardiac failure (Fig. 65b). Check for ascites, pleural effusions, and dilated inferior vena cava and hepatic veins (see pp. 68 and 76). Examine the patient.

5. Chronic renal insufficiency. Examine the kidneys and the urine.

6. Multiple myeloma. Laboratory tests are necessary.

7. Hyperplastic cholecystosis. This is usually asymptomatic. Aschoff-Rokitansky sinuses are best seen on oral cholecystography, occasionally with ultrasound.

8. Acute hepatitis.

9. Lymphoma.

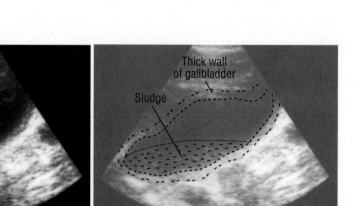

Fig. 65a. A gallbladder with thick walls due to chronic cholecystitis: the bile is thickened, forming sludge.

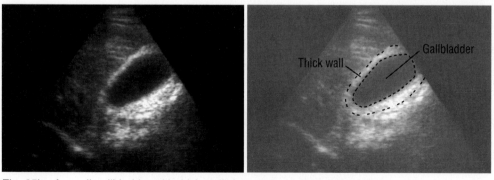

Fig. 65b. A small gallbladder with thick walls in a patient with cardiac failure.

Localized thickening

Local thickening of the gallbladder walls may be due to the following:

1. Mucosal folds. There may be several together. Scan in different positions: pathological thickening (more than 5 mm in any area) will not alter with the position of the patient, but folds will vary in thickness and position (Fig. 65c).

2. Polyp. There will be no movement with a change in the patient's position (Fig. 65d), but the shape may alter.

3. Primary or secondary carcinoma of the gallbladder. This appears as a thick, irregular, solid intramural mass, localized and not changing with the patient's position (Fig. 65e).

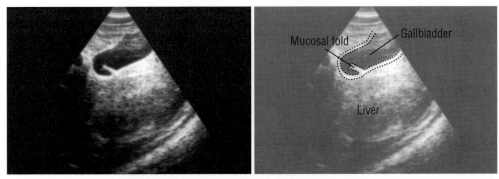

Fig. 65c. A mucosal fold in the gallbladder. Rescanning in different positions, or after an interval, is essential to establish the correct diagnosis.

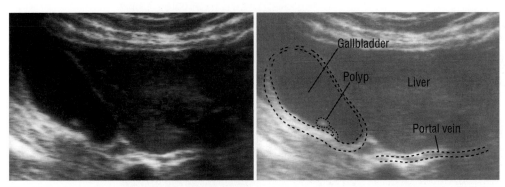

Fig. 65d. A small pedunculated polyp. This will not move but may alter its shape when the patient is scanned in a different position.

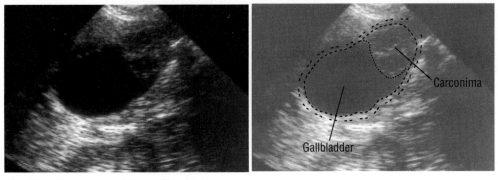

Fig. 65e. Carcinoma of the gallbladder.

Small gallbladder

1. The patient may recently have had a meal containing fat and the gallbladder has contracted.

2. Chronic cholecystitis: check for thickened gallbladder walls and for gallstones within the gallbladder (Fig. 66a) (see pp. 100–102).

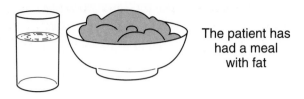

The patient has had a meal with fat

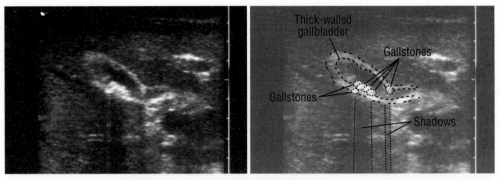

Fig. 66a. A small thick-walled gallbladder containing several stones.

If the gallbladder is small, re-examine after 6–8 hours (without food or drink) to differentiate between an empty gallbladder and a contracted gallbladder. The normal gallbladder will fill up after a few hours and appear normal in size.

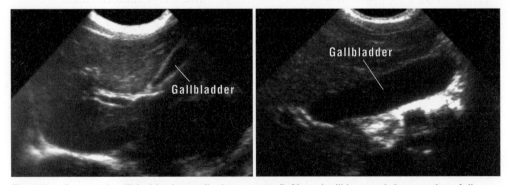

Fig. 66b. A normal gallbladder is small when empty (left) and will be much larger when full (right).

Jaundice

When the patient is jaundiced, ultrasound can usually differentiate between non-obstructive and obstructive jaundice, by showing the dilatation of the biliary system. *However, the exact cause of the jaundice may be difficult to identify.*

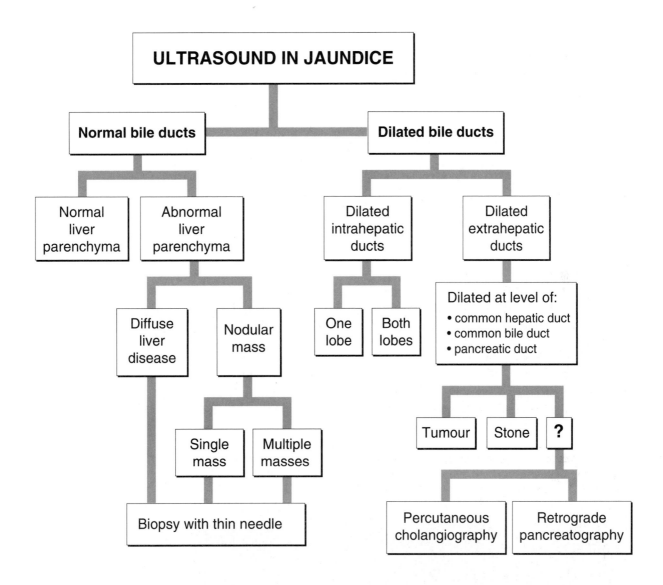

When the patient is jaundiced, ultrasound can provide information about the gallbladder and the biliary ducts, and can usually differentiate between obstructive and non-obstructive jaundice, but does not always show the exact cause.

In every jaundiced patient, scan the liver, the biliary tract and both sides of the upper abdomen.

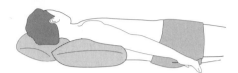

Technique

The patient should be supine, with the right side slightly elevated. Ask the patient to take a deep breath and hold it in while the scan is being performed.

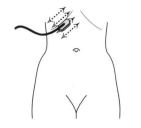

For an adult, use a 3.5 MHz transducer. For a child or thin adult, use a 5 MHz transducer.

Start with sagittal or slightly oblique scans; identify the inferior vena cava and the main portal vein lying anteriorly. This will make it easier to locate the common hepatic duct and the common bile duct, which should be seen angling from the liver anteriorly to the portal vein and descending to the pancreas (Fig. 59) (see p. 96).

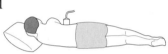

In one-third of patients, the bile duct will be more lateral to the portal vein and is better seen by oblique longitudinal scanning (Fig. 67a).

Normal bile ducts

1. Extrahepatic ducts. It may be difficult to see the extrahepatic bile ducts, particularly with a linear transducer. Use a curvilinear or sector transducer if available. Move the patient into different positions, varying the scanning technique as much as possible whenever the extrahepatic duct needs to be demonstrated (Fig. 67a).

2. Intrahepatic ducts. The intrahepatic ducts are best seen on the left side of the liver in deep inspiration (Fig. 67b). It is not easy to see the normal intrahepatic ducts on ultrasound because they are often too small and thin-walled. However, *when the ducts are dilated, they are easily seen* and show as numerous, branching irregular structures throughout the liver substance (the "branching tree" effect) near the portal veins (Fig. 67b).

3.5 MHz   5 MHz
adults   children

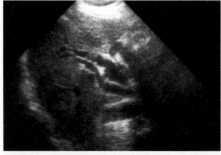 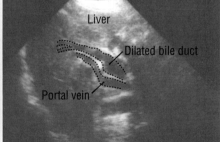

Fig. 67a. Dilated extrahepatic bile ducts.

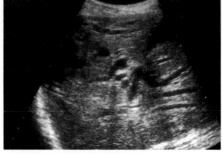 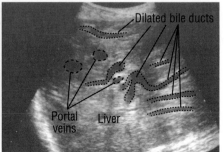

Fig. 67b. Dilated intrahepatic bile ducts.

Gallbladder in jaundice

1. If the gallbladder is distended, the obstruction usually affects the common bile duct (e.g. calculus, *Ascaris*, acute pancreatitis or carcinoma). The hepatic ducts will also be distended (Fig. 68a).

2. If the gallbladder is not distended or is very small Fig. 68b), obstruction is unlikely or the obstruction is above the level of the cystic duct (e.g. enlarged lymph nodes or tumour near the porta hepatis).

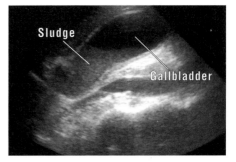

Fig. 68a. A distended gallbladder.

Biliary tract in jaundice

- **Maximum diameter of normal common hepatic duct: less than 5 mm**

- **Maximum diameter of normal common bile duct: less than 9 mm**

- **Maximum diameter of common bile duct post-cholecystectomy: 10–12 mm**

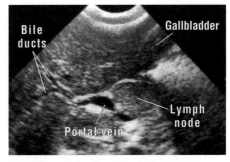

Fig. 68b. A small gallbladder with distended bile ducts (due to an enlarged lymph node at the porta hepatis).

Sometimes following surgery, and in patients over 70 years of age, the common bile duct may be a few millimetres wider (i.e. 12–14 mm) (Fig. 68c). Add 1 mm to all of the measurements above for each decade over 70 years of age.

1. If the intrahepatic ducts are mildly dilated, suspect biliary obstruction which can be recognized on ultrasound before there is clinical jaundice (Fig. 68d).

   If in the early stages of jaundice the bile ducts are not dilated, rescan after 24 hours.

2. If the extrahepatic ducts are dilated, but not the intra-hepatic ducts, scan the liver parenchyma. If jaundice is persistent, the cause may be cirrhosis. But also exclude obstruction of the lower common bile duct (Fig. 68e).

Dilated intrahepatic ducts are best seen by scanning the sub-xiphoid region to show the left lobe of the liver. They will appear as tubular structures parallel to the portal vein, both centrally and extending into the periphery of the liver.

If it seems that there are two vessels running parallel, one is most likely a dilated bile duct, which will also be seen extending elsewhere in the liver, probably about the same size as the portal veins.

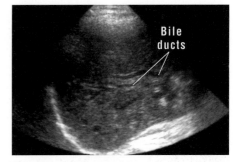

Fig. 68c. Mildly dilated bile ducts.

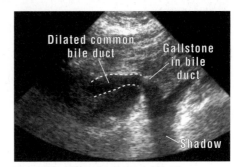

Fig. 68d. Dilated common bile duct containing a gallstone.

Clonorchiasis

In clonorchiasis, the common and hepatic bile ducts are dilated, irregular and saccular, whereas in obstructive jaundice without cholangitis, the ducts are smoothly dilated and seldom saccular. It is possible to recognize intraductal debris in clonorchiasis but the actual parasites are too small to be imaged with ultrasound (Fig. 69).

If both the hepatic and extrahepatic bile ducts are dilated and there are large cystic lesions within the liver parenchyma, there is probably hydatid disease, not clonorchiasis (see pp. 82–83).

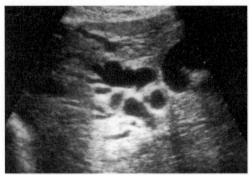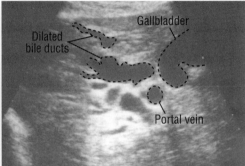

Fig. 69a. Longitudinal scan: dilated and irregular bile ducts due to infective cholangitis, often associated with clonorchiasis.

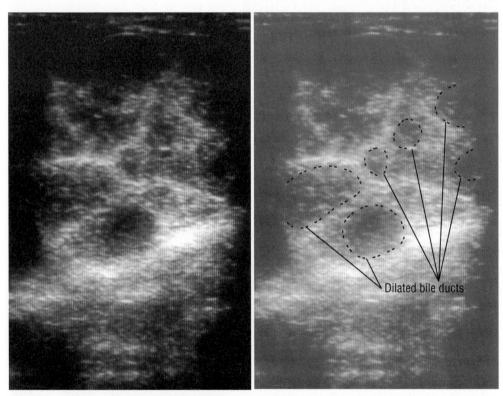

Fig. 69b. Transverse scan: dilated, saccular bile ducts filled with debris from infection. Gross distension such as this is found in clonorchiasis.

Ultrasound can diagnose gallstones in the gallbladder but is not always reliable in recognizing stones in the common bile duct. Clinical judgement must be used, especially in the jaundiced patient.

CHAPTER 10

Pancreas

Indications

1. Midline upper abdominal pain, acute or chronic.
2. Jaundice.
3. Upper abdominal mass.
4. Persistent fever, especially with upper abdominal tenderness.
5. Suspected malignant disease.
6. Recurrent chronic pancreatitis.
7. Suspected complications of acute pancreatitis, especially pseudocyst or abscess.
8. Polycystic kidneys: cysts in the liver or spleen.
9. Direct abdominal trauma, particularly in children.

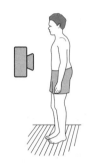

If there is acute abdominal pain, an erect radiograph of the upper abdomen, including both sides of the diaphragm, is needed to exclude perforation of a hollow viscus.

Preparation

1. **Preparation of the patient**. The patient should take *nothing* by mouth for 8 hours preceding the examination. If fluid is essential to prevent dehydration, only water should be given. If the symptoms are acute, proceed with the examination. Infants—clinical condition permitting—should be given *nothing* by mouth for 3 hours preceding the examination.

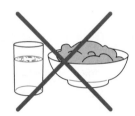

2. **Position of the patient.** The patient should be supine but may need to be examined in the oblique or both decubitus positions: if necessary, a scan can be done with the patient sitting partially upright or in the erect position.

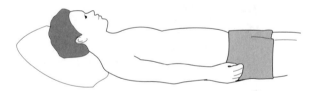

    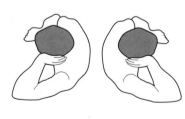   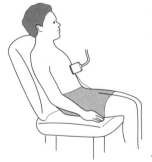   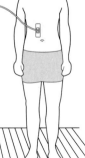

oblique   decubitus

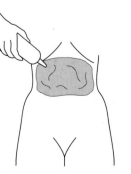

Apply coupling agent liberally across the upper abdomen on both sides.

3. **Choice of transducer.** Use a 3.5 MHz transducer for adults. Use a 5 MHz transducer for children or thin adults.

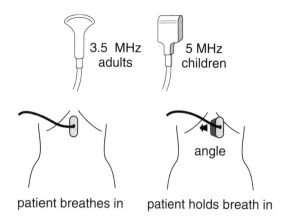

4. **Setting the correct gain**. Start by placing the transducer centrally at the top of the abdomen (the xiphoid angle).

   Angle the beam to the right side of the patient to image the liver; adjust the gain to obtain the best image (see p. 50).

Scanning technique

The pancreas can be *very* difficult to identify, especially the tail.

Start with transverse upper abdominal scans moving from side to side and from the costal margin towards the umbilicus. Then perform longitudinal scans moving up and down across the upper abdomen. When it is necessary to examine a specific area, ask the patient to take a deep breath and hold it in.

Gas

If bowel gas obscures the image:

1. Try gentle compression with the transducer or use decubitus views, both right and left.

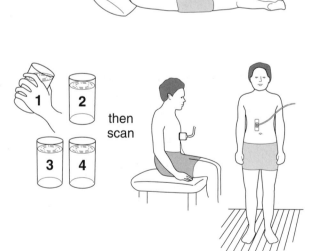

2. If necessary, give the patient 3 or 4 glasses of water, wait a few minutes to allow the bubbles to disperse and then repeat the examination with the patient sitting or standing, viewing the pancreas through the water-filled stomach.

3. If the patient cannot stand, let him or her lie on the left side and drink through a straw. Then scan with the patient supine (see also p. 116).

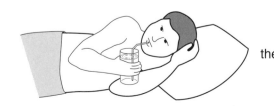

then scan

Transverse scanning

Start with transverse scans across the abdomen moving downwards towards the feet until the splenic vein is seen as a linear, tubular structure with the medial end broadened. This is where it is joined by the superior mesenteric vein, at the level of the body of the pancreas. The superior mesenteric artery will be seen in cross-section just below the vein. By angling and rocking the transducer, the head and the tail of the pancreas may be seen (Fig. 70).

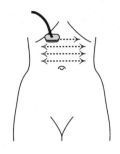

Continue transverse scans downwards to visualize the head of the pancreas and the uncinate process (if present) between the inferior vena cava and the portal vein (Fig. 70a).

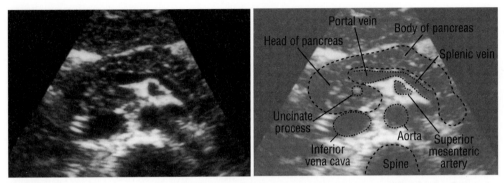

Fig. 70a. Transverse scan: the splenic vein, superior mesenteric artery and the body of the pancreas.

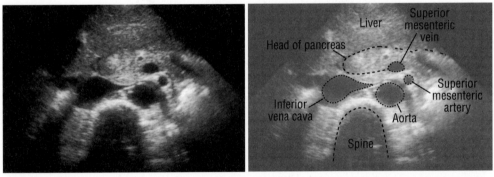

Fig. 70b. Transverse scan: the head of a normal pancreas scanned through the left lobe of the liver.

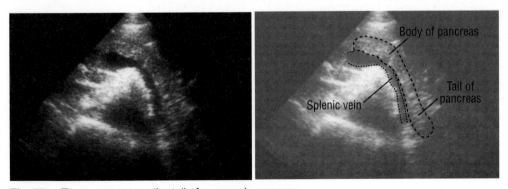

Fig. 70c. Transverse scan: the tail of a normal pancreas.

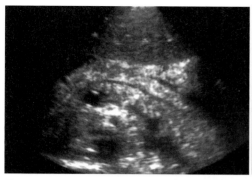
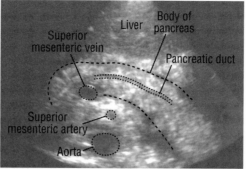
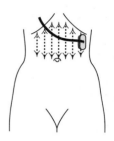
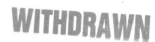

Fig. 70d. Transverse scan: the normal pancreatic duct.

Longitudinal scanning

Start longitudinal scanning just to the right of the midline and identify the tubular pattern of the inferior vena cava with the head of the pancreas anteriorly, below the liver. The vena cava should not be compressed or flattened by a normal pancreas (Fig. 71a).

Continue longitudinal scans moving to the left. Identify the aorta and the superior mesenteric artery. This will assist in identifying the body of the pancreas (Fig. 71b).

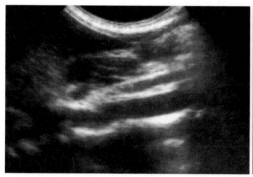
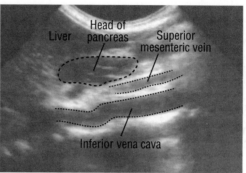

Fig. 71a. Longitudinal scan: the inferior vena cava and the head of the pancreas.

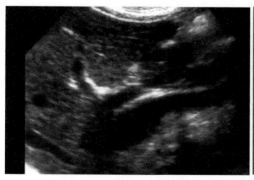
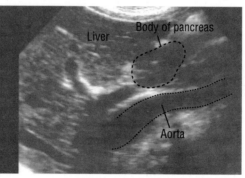

Fig. 71b. Longitudinal scan: the body of the pancreas.

Decubitus scanning

After the transverse and longitudinal scans, turn the patient onto the right side and scan the pancreas through the spleen and the left kidney. This will demonstrate the tail of the pancreas.

Then, with the patient lying on the left side, ask him/her to take a deep breath and hold it in. Scan the pancreas through the liver. This will show the head of the pancreas (Fig. 72).

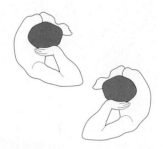

full inspiration

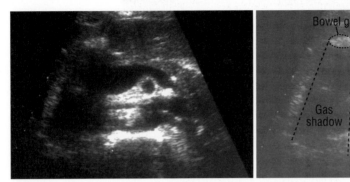

Fig. 72a. The head of the pancreas is obscured by bowel gas when the patient is supine.

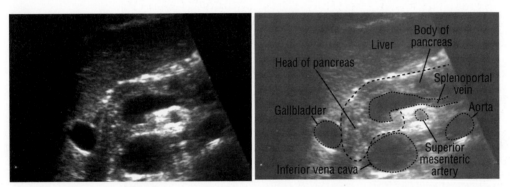

Fig. 72b. When the same patient is in the left decubitus position, the bowel gas has moved and the pancreas is seen clearly.

Erect scanning

When visualization is poor because of bowel gas, let the patient drink 3 or 4 glasses of water. Once the patient has finished drinking wait a few minutes for the bubbles to disperse. Then, with the patient sitting or erect, scan the pancreas through the stomach. This technique is particularly useful for visualizing the tail of the pancreas (Fig. 72c, d) (see also p. 113).

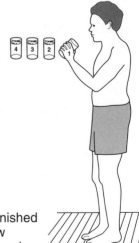

After patient has finished drinking, wait a few minutes before scanning

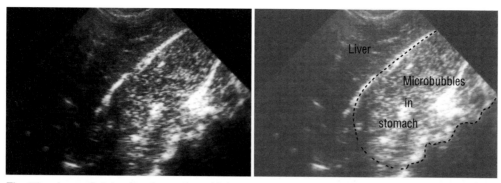

Fig. 72c. Immediately after the patient drinks water, wait before scanning. Microbubbles in the stomach may obscure the pancreas.

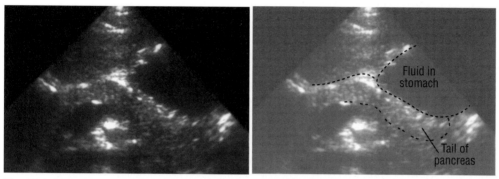

Fig. 72d. With the patient erect, the pancreas can be scanned through the stomach.

Imaging the entire pancreas is often difficult. Different positions and scanning angles must be used.

Normal pancreas

The pancreas has about the same echogenicity as the adjacent liver and should appear homogeneous. However, the pancreatic echogenicity increases with age. The outline of the normal pancreas is smooth.

When scanning the pancreas, certain anatomical landmarks should be identified, in the following order:

1. Aorta
2. Inferior vena cava
3. Superior mesenteric artery
4. Splenic vein
5. Superior mesenteric vein
6. Wall of the stomach
7. Common bile duct

The *essential* landmarks are the superior mesenteric artery and the splenic vein.

Normal pancreatic size

There is great variability in the size and shape of the pancreas. The following guidelines may be helpful.

1. The average diameter of the head of the pancreas (A): 2.8 cm.

2. The average diameter of the medial part of the body of the pancreas (B): less than 2 cm.

3. The average diameter of the tail of the pancreas (C): 2.5 cm.

4. The diameter of the pancreatic duct should not exceed 2 mm. It is normally smooth, and the wall and the lumen can be identified. The accessory pancreatic duct is seldom visualized.

Fat patient

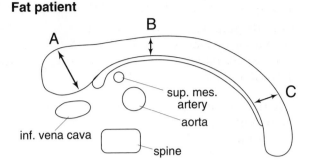

Thin patient

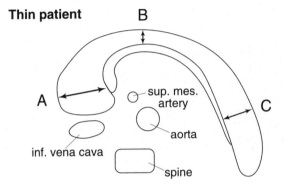

Small pancreas

The pancreas is usually smaller in elderly people, but this is not of clinical significance. When there is overall atrophy of the pancreas, the decrease in size is usually uniform throughout the pancreas. If there appears to be atrophy of the tail of the pancreas alone (the head appearing normal), then a tumour in the head of the pancreas must be suspected (Fig. 73a). The head must be scanned carefully because chronic pancreatitis in the body and tail may be associated with a slow-growing tumour in the head of the pancreas.

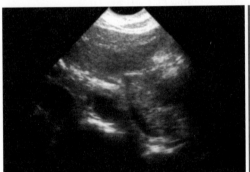
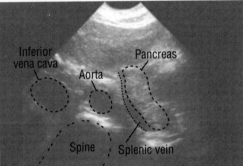

Fig. 73a. Atrophy of the tail of the pancreas.

If the pancreas is small and irregularly hyperechogenic and non-homogeneous compared with the liver, the cause is usually chronic pancreatitis (Fig. 73b).

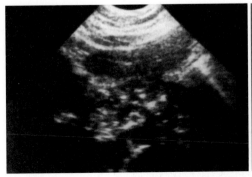
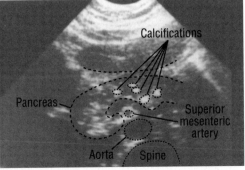

Fig. 73b. A small, nonhomogeneous pancreas with calcifications due to chronic pancreatitis.

Diffuse enlargement of the pancreas

In acute pancreatitis, the pancreas may be diffusely enlarged and either normal or hypoechogenic compared with the adjacent liver. The serum amylase is usually elevated, and there may be local ileus due to bowel irritation.

When the pancreas is irregularly hyperechogenic and diffusely enlarged, there is usually acute pancreatitis superimposed on chronic pancreatitis (Fig. 74a).

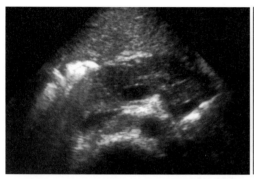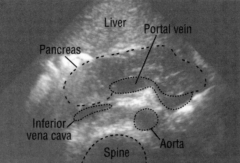

Fig. 74a. Transverse scan: acute pancreatitis.

Focal enlargement (noncystic)

Almost all pancreatic tumours are hypoechogenic compared with the normal pancreas. It is not possible to distinguish between focal pancreatitis or pancreatic tumour by ultrasound alone. Even if the serum amylase is elevated, repeat the ultrasound examination in 2 weeks to assess the change. Tumour and pancreatitis can co-exist. When the pattern is mixed, biopsy is needed (Fig. 74b).

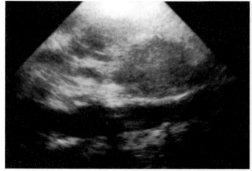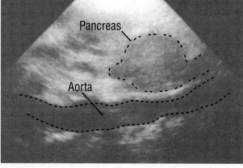

Fig. 74b. Longitudinal scan: focal, noncystic enlargement of the pancreas due to chronic pancreatitis. A tumour could have the same appearance.

	Tumour	Acute pancreatitis, diffuse or local	Chronic pancreatitis	Aging normal pancreas
Echogenicity relative to the adjacent liver	Low	Low	High	High

Ultrasound cannot distinguish focal pancreatitis from a pancreatic tumour.

Pancreatic cysts

True pancreatic cysts are rare. They are usually single, echo-free, smooth cavities filled with fluid. Small multiple cysts may be congenital. An abscess or haematoma in the pancreas will appear as a complex mass, often associated with severe pancreatitis.

Pseudocysts following trauma or acute pancreatitis are not uncommon; they may increase in size and rupture. Such cysts can be single or multiple. In the early stages they are complex, with internal echoes and ill-defined walls, but eventually these cysts become smooth-walled and echo-free, with good sound transmission (Fig. 75a). Pancreatic pseudocysts may be found anywhere in the abdomen or pelvis, often remote from the pancreas. When the cysts are infected or damaged, there may be internal echoes or septation.

Pancreatic cystadenoma or other cystic tumours usually appear on ultrasound as multiseptate cystic masses with associated solid components (Fig. 75b). In microcysticadenomata the cysts are very small and difficult to image.

Hydatid cysts (Fig. 75c) are unusual in the pancreas. Scan the liver and the rest of the abdomen to exclude hydatid disease (see pp. 82–83).

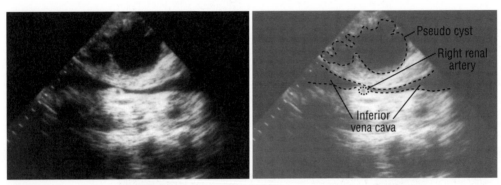

Fig. 75a. Longitudinal scan: a pseudocyst of the pancreas.

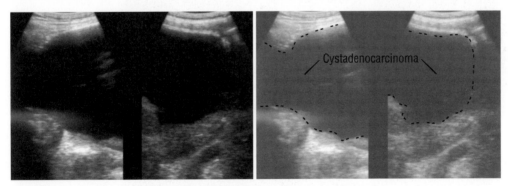

Fig. 75b. Longitudinal scans: cystadenocarcinoma of the pancreas.

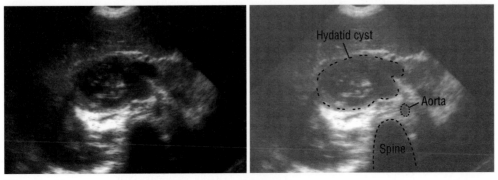

Fig. 75c. Transverse scan: hydatid cyst of the pancreas.

Calcification in the pancreas

Ultrasound is not the best way to assess pancreatic calcification. A supine antero–posterior radiograph of the upper abdomen is preferable.

Calcification within the pancreas can produce acoustic shadowing. However, if the calcification is very small, there may only be bright discrete echoes without shadowing. Calcification is usually due to:

1. Chronic pancreatitis. Calcification is distributed throughout the pancreas (Fig. 76a, b).

2. Calculi in the pancreatic duct. This calcification follows the anatomical pattern of the duct (Fig. 76c).

3. Biliary calculi in the distal common bile duct can be mistaken for pancreatic calcification. There is usually dilatation of the proximal bile duct.

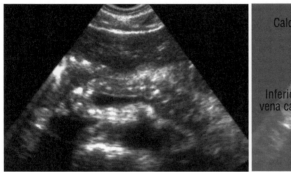
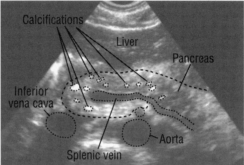

Fig. 76a. Chronic pancreatitis with calcification.

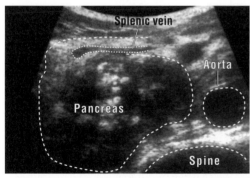
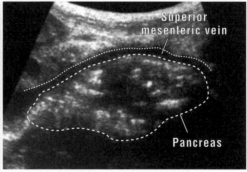

Fig. 76b. Transverse (left) and longitudinal (right) scans of chronic pancreatitis with calcification.

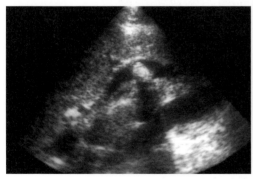
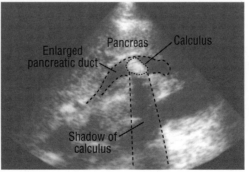

Fig. 76c. Transverse scan: a large calculus in the pancreatic duct.

Dilatation of the pancreatic duct

The normal maximum internal diameter of the pancreatic duct is 2 mm, and it is best identified on a transverse scan of the mid portion of the body of the pancreas. To ensure proper identification of the duct, pancreatic tissue should be recognized on either side of it. If not, either the splenic vein posteriorly or the wall of the stomach anteriorly may cause confusion (Fig. 77a).

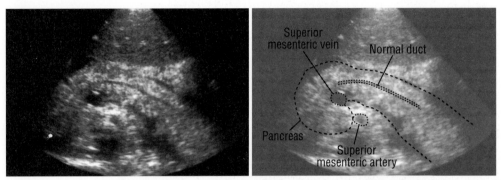

Fig. 77a. The internal diameter of a normal pancreatic duct should be less than 2 mm.

The walls of the pancreatic duct should be smooth and the lumen clear. When the duct is dilated, the walls become irregular; scan not only the head of the pancreas but also the biliary tract (Fig. 77b).

The causes of dilatation of the pancreatic duct are:

1. Tumour of the head of the pancreas or of the ampulla of Vater. Both are usually associated with jaundice and dilatation of the biliary tract.

2. Calculus in the common pancreatic duct. Scan to visualize biliary calculi and bile duct dilatation (see pp. 96 and 107–109).

3. Calculus in the intrapancreatic duct. The biliary tract should be normal.

4. Chronic pancreatitis (see pp. 118–119 and 121).

5. Postoperative strictures following Whipple's operation or partial pancreatectomy. The clinical history should be verified with the patient or relatives if necessary.

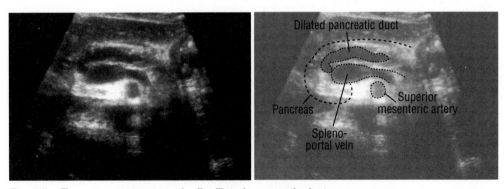

Fig. 77b. Transverse scan: a markedly dilated pancreatic duct.

Common errors: when scanning the pancreas, an incorrect diagnosis may be made because:

- The gallbladder is in the midline.

- There are enlarged lymph nodes.

- There is a retroperitoneal mass.

- There is loculated ascites or an intra-abdominal abscess (including splenic abscess).

- There are hepatic cysts or tumours.

- There are mesenteric cysts.

- There is a haematoma around the duodenum.

- The stomach is partially filled. If the stomach contains fluid, it may resemble a pancreatic cyst; if it contains food, it may mimic a tumour. The adjacent bowel can cause similar errors.

- There are renal cysts, a renal tumour or a large renal pelvis.

- There is an aortic aneurysm.

- There is an adrenal tumour.

Notes

CHAPTER 11

Spleen

Indications

1. Splenomegaly (enlarged spleen)

2. Left abdominal mass

3. Blunt abdominal trauma

4. Left upper abdominal pain (an erect abdominal X-ray, including both sides of the diaphragm, is also needed if perforation of the bowel is suspected)

5. Suspected subphrenic abscess (pyrexia of unknown origin)

6. Jaundice combined with anaemia

7. Echinococcosis (hydatid disease)

8. Ascites or localized intra-abdominal fluid

9. Suspected malignancy, especially lymphoma or leukaemia

Preparation

1. **Preparation of the patient**. The patient should take *nothing* by mouth for 8 hours preceding the examination. If fluid is essential to prevent dehydration, only water should be given. If the symptoms are acute, proceed with the examination. Infants—clinical condition permitting—should be given *nothing* by mouth for 3 hours preceding the examination.

   For acutely ill patients (e.g. trauma, sudden abdominal pain, post-surgical pyrexia), no preparation is needed.

2. **Position of the patient**. The patient should be supine initially and later on the right side.

   Apply coupling agent liberally over the left lower chest, the upper abdomen and left flank.

   The patient should take a deep breath and hold it in when a specific area is being scanned.

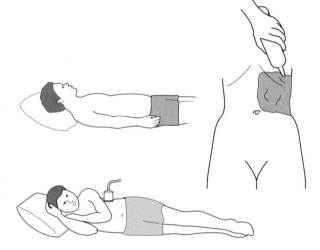

3. **Choice of transducer**. For adults, use a 3.5 MHz sector transducer. For children and thin adults, use a 5 MHz sector transducer. A small sector transducer is helpful, if available.

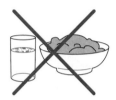

3.5 MHz
adults

5 MHz
children

4. **Setting the correct gain**. Start by placing the transducer centrally at the top of the abdomen (the xiphoid angle). Angle the beam to the right side of the patient to image the liver; adjust the gain to obtain the best image (see p. 50).

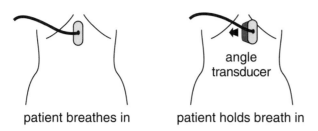

patient breathes in   patient holds breath in

Scanning technique

Scan with the patient in the supine and oblique positions. Multiple scans may be necessary.

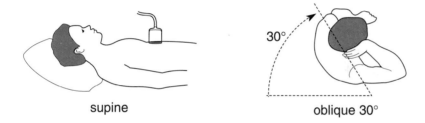

supine   oblique 30°

Scan from below the costal margin, angling the beam towards the diaphragm, then in the ninth intercostal space downwards. Repeat through all lower intercostal spaces, first with the patient supine and then with the patient lying obliquely (30°) on the right side.

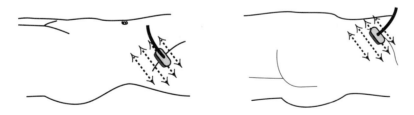

Also perform longitudinal scans from anterior to posterior axillary lines and transverse upper abdominal scans. Scan the liver also, particularly when the spleen is enlarged.

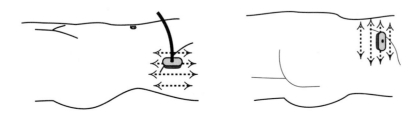

Normal spleen

It is important to identify the:

1. Left hemi-diaphragm.
2. Splenic hilus.
3. Splenic veins and relationship to pancreas.
4. Left kidney (and renal/splenic relationship).
5. Left edge of liver.
6. Pancreas.

When the spleen is normal in size, it can be difficult to image completely. The splenic hilus is the reference point to ensure correct identification of the spleen. Identify the hilus as the entry point for the splenic vessels (Fig. 78).

> **It is important to identify the left diaphragm and the upper edge of the spleen.**

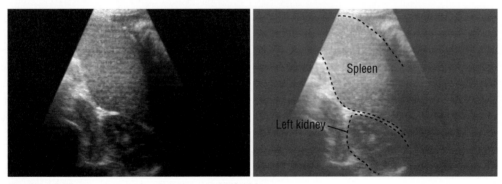

Fig. 78. Oblique scan: normal spleen and left kidney.

Echo pattern

The spleen should show a uniform homogeneous echo pattern. It is slightly less echogenic than the liver.

Echogenicity

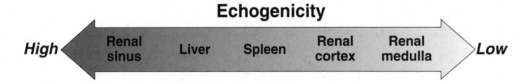

High ◄ Renal sinus | Liver | Spleen | Renal cortex | Renal medulla ► Low

> ## Common errors in scanning the spleen
>
> **The following may be mistaken for splenic lesions:**
>
> • **A kidney lesion.**
>
> • **The tail of the pancreas.**
>
> • **Adrenal tumours.**
>
> • **The stomach.**
>
> **Identify these organs before looking at the spleen.**

Abnormal spleen

Enlarged spleen/splenomegaly

There are no absolute criteria for the size of the spleen on ultrasound. When normal, it is a little larger than or about the same size as the left kidney. The length should not exceed 15 cm in the major axis.

A chronically enlarged spleen may often distort and displace the left kidney, narrowing it in both the antero–posterior diameter and the width.

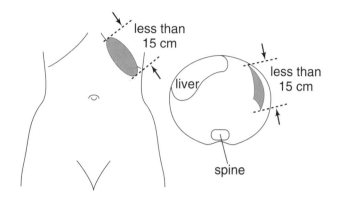

Homogeneous splenomegaly

This may be due to:

1. Tropical splenomegaly, which includes idiopathic splenomegaly, malaria, trypanosomiasis, leishmaniasis and schistosomiasis (Fig. 79a).
2. Sickle cell disease (unless infarcted).
3. Portal hypertension.
4. Leukaemia (Fig. 79b).
4. Metabolic disease.
5. Lymphoma (may contain hyperechogenic masses).
6. Infections such as rubella and mononucleosis.

Whenever there is splenomegaly, examine the liver for size and echogenicity. Also examine the splenic and portal veins, the inferior vena cava, hepatic veins and mesentery for thickening. The region near the hilum of the spleen should be scanned for tubular structures due to varicosities.

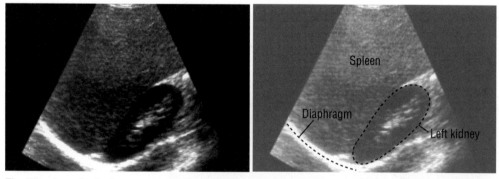

Fig. 79a. Longitudinal scan: gross splenomegaly (due to leishmaniasis) compressing the left kidney.

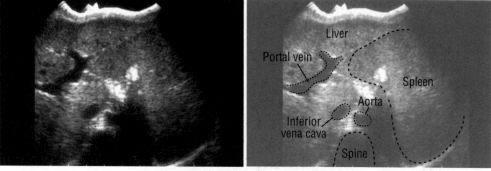

Fig. 79b. Transverse scan: hepatosplenomegaly due to leukaemia.

Non-homogeneous spleen, with or without splenomegaly

Well defined cystic lesion

If there is a clearly demarcated, echo-free mass with posterior acoustic enhancement, differentiate:

1. **Cystic disease** (may be multiple). Examine liver and pancreas for cysts.

2. **Congenital cysts**. These are usually solitary and may contain echoes as a result of haemorrhage (Fig. 80a).

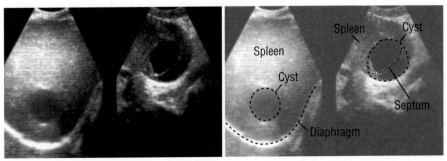

Fig. 80a. Longitudinal scans: a septate cyst in the spleen, found incidentally.

3. **Echinococcal (hydatid) cysts**. These are usually clearly defined with a double wall (the pericyst and the cyst wall) and often septate. There will be markedly enhanced back wall echoes and often marked variation in the thickness of the wall of the cyst. However, hydatid cysts may appear as roughly rounded masses with an irregular contour and a mixed echo pattern resembling an abscess. The cyst can be hypoechogenic with few irregular echoes or hyperechogenic and solid without any back wall shadow: combinations of these findings may occur. The walls of the cyst may be collapsed or sagging and there may be a floating density within the cyst, or even a cyst within a cyst (which is pathognomonic for hydatid disease). There may be calcification within the wall of the cyst and there may be "sand" in the most dependent portion. Examine the whole abdomen and X-ray the chest. Hydatid cysts are often multiple but the pattern is variable and cysts in the liver do not always resemble those in the spleen (Fig. 80b) (see pp. 82–83 and 135).

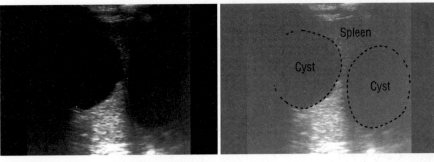

Fig. 80b. Hydatid cysts in the spleen.

4. **Haematoma**. See p. 134.

> **If the spleen is enlarged, and there is a history of trauma, scan the spleen to exclude injury (see p. 134).**

A regular but ill-defined cystic lesion in the spleen

Scan in different projections.

1. A hypoechogenic cystic area with an irregular outline, usually containing debris and associated with splenomegaly and local tenderness, suggests a splenic abscess (Fig. 81a). Examine the liver for other abscesses (see pp. 78 and 86–87).

   After successful treatment, the abscess may resolve or become larger and almost echo-free, but is no longer tender (Fig. 81b).

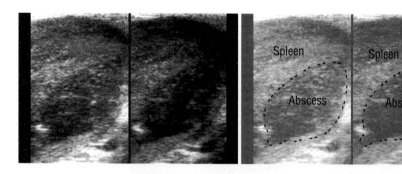

Fig. 81a. An early abscess in the spleen, before treatment.

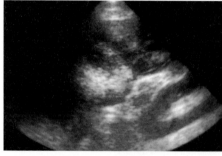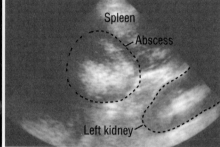

Fig. 81b. A splenic abscess after treatment.

2. A similar cystic lesion which is larger and contains fluid may be a splenic abscess following infarction resulting from sickle cell disease. Amoebic abscesses are very rare in the spleen: bacterial abscesses are more common.

Splenic vein

A normal splenic vein does not exclude portal hypertension.

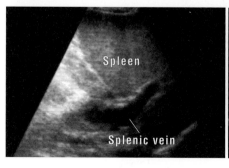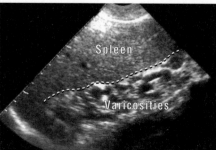

Fig. 81c. Two patients with dilatation of the splenic vein and multiple varicosities, the results of portal hypertension.

Enlarged splenic vein

If the splenic vein appears large and remains more than 10 mm in diameter on normal respiration, portal hypertension should be suspected. When the portal vein is more than 13 mm in diameter and does not vary with respiration, there is a strong correlation with portal hypertension (Fig. 81c).

Intrasplenic mass, with or without splenomegaly

Splenic masses may be single or multiple and well defined or irregular in outline. Lymphoma is the commonest cause of an intrasplenic mass, and such masses are usually hypoechogenic (Fig. 82a). Malignant tumours, either primary or metastatic, are rare and may be either hypo- or hyperechogenic (Fig. 82b). When there is necrosis there will be a complex echo pattern, which may suggest an abscess (Fig. 82d, p. 133). Infections such as tuberculosis or histoplasmosis may cause scattered granulomas, appearing as hyperechogenic masses, sometimes with shadowing because of calcification. Haematoma must be excluded (see pp. 134–135).

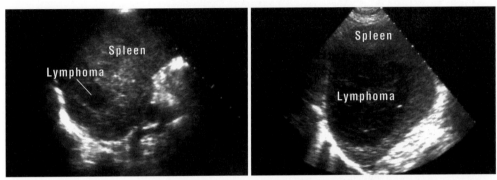

Fig. 82a. Two patients with lymphoma of the spleen: a small mass in the spleen on the left, a much larger mass in the spleen on the right. Both masses are hypoechogenic.

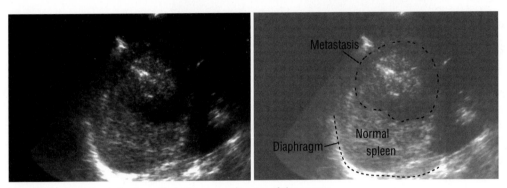

Fig. 82b. Metastasis in the spleen from carcinoma of the ovary.

If there is contraction of the splenic outline near the mass, there may be an old haematoma or scar from trauma (see pp. 134–135). Alternatively, there may be an old infarct (e.g. in sickle cell disease) (Fig. 82c).

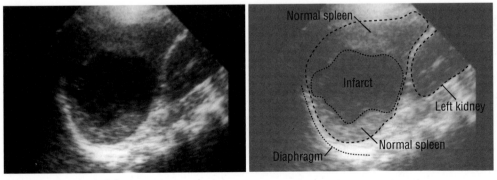

Fig. 82c. A splenic infarct.

Whenever there is an intrasplenic mass, exclude recent injury, particularly when there is splenomegaly.

Splenic abscess: an irregular, hypoechogenic or complex cystic intrasplenic mass (Fig. 82d). See also pp. 131–132.

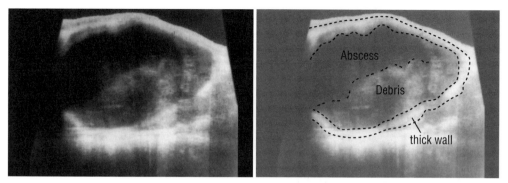

Fig. 82d. A large splenic abscess, containing debris and almost filling the spleen.

Pyrexia (usually of unknown origin)

If possible, check the total and the differential white cell count. Start with longitudinal scans.

A perisplenic, subdiaphragmatic, echo-free or complex mass, superior to the spleen but limited by the left diaphragm, is probably a subphrenic abscess. Movement of the diaphragm will usually be reduced. Scan under the right diaphragm to see if there is fluid on that side. Also scan the whole abdomen, including the pelvis, to exclude fluid elsewhere. Scan the left lateral and posterior lower chest for an echo-free area above the diaphragm indicating pleural fluid, sometimes visible through the spleen (Fig. 83). A chest X-ray may be helpful.

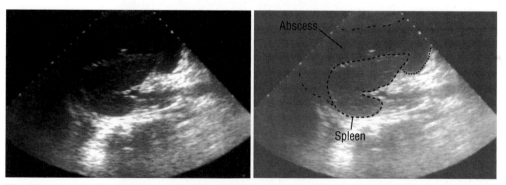

Fig. 83a. Longitudinal scan: a collection of fluid around the spleen; this was a perisplenic abscess, but the type of fluid can seldom be identified with an ultrasound scan.

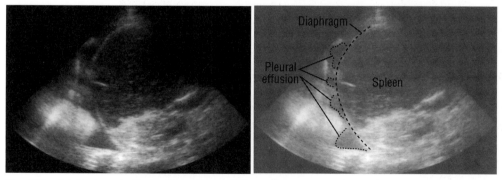

Fig. 83b. A left pleural effusion seen through the spleen.

Trauma

The examination should include a survey of the outline of the spleen, to identify any area of local enlargement, and then the abdomen to determine the presence or absence of free intraperitoneal fluid. Repeat the scan after a few days if the clinical condition of the patient is not improving.

1. If there is free intraperitoneal or subphrenic fluid and an irregular splenic outline, a splenic tear or injury is likely (Fig. 84a, b).

2. An echo-free or complex echo area at the periphery of the spleen, associated with general or localized splenomegaly suggests a subcapsular haematoma (Fig. 84c). Search carefully for free intra-abdominal fluid.

3. An intrasplenic echo-free or complex, irregular mass suggests an acute haematoma (Fig. 84d). An accessory spleen may have the same appearance (Fig. 84e).

4. An echogenic intrasplenic mass is probably an old haematoma which has calcified, giving bright echoes with acoustic shadowing. A haemangioma may have the same appearance (Fig. 84f).

5. An irregular, echo-free or complex mass may be a traumatic cyst or a damaged hydatid cyst (Fig. 84g) (see p. 130).

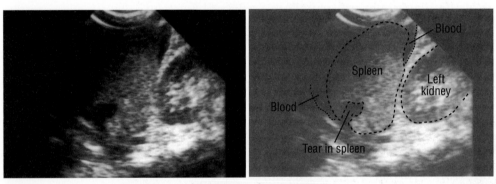

Fig. 84a. A tear in the upper pole of the spleen following injury.

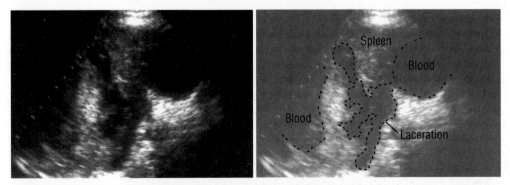

Fig. 84b. Laceration of the spleen with intra-abdominal fluid, probably blood.

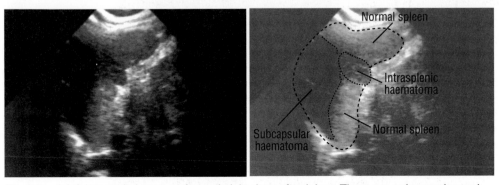

Fig. 84c. A left intercostal scan performed eight days after injury. There are subcapsular and intrasplenic haematomas.

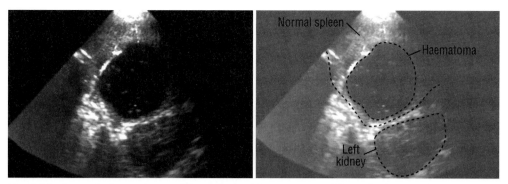

Fig. 84d. An acute haematoma of the spleen without rupture of the splenic capsule.

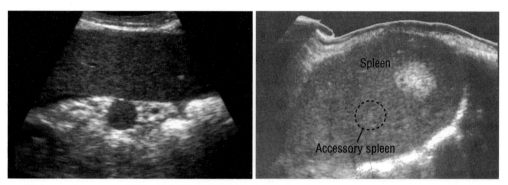

Fig. 84e. An accessory spleen: this could be mistaken for a haematoma or the result of a torn spleen.

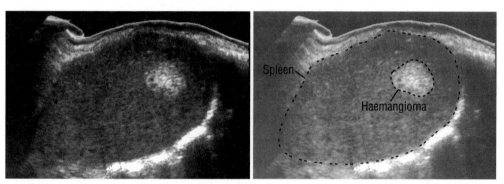

Fig. 84f. An enlarged spleen due to tropical splenomegaly, in which a solitary haemangioma was an incidental finding. It could be mistaken for an old haematoma or a collapsed cyst.

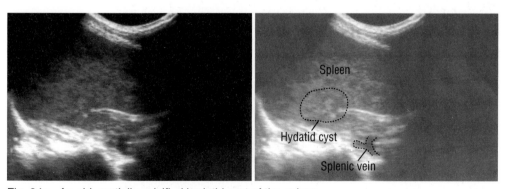

Fig. 84g. An old, partially calcified hydatid cyst of the spleen.

If there is a history of trauma to the abdomen within the previous 10 days, suspect damage to the spleen when there is splenomegaly, persistent anaemia or intra-abdominal fluid.

136

Notes

CHAPTER 12

Peritoneal cavity and gastrointestinal tract

Indications

In adults

1. Suspected ascites and peritonitis
2. Abdominal mass
3. Suspected appendicitis (particularly to exclude other conditions)
4. Localized abdominal pain

In children

1. Localized pain and abdominal masses
2. Suspected hypertrophic pyloric stenosis
3. Suspected intussusception
4. Suspected but indeterminate appendicitis
5. Ascites and peritonitis

Preparation

1. **Preparation of the patient**. The patient should take *nothing* by mouth for 8 hours preceding the examination. If fluid is desirable, only water should be given. If the symptoms are acute, proceed with the examination.

   Infants—clinical condition permitting—should be given *nothing* by mouth for 3–4 hours preceding the examination. If the child is vomiting and suspected of having hypertrophic pyloric stenosis, a warm, sweet, non-aerated drink is necessary to fill the stomach so that it is possible to check for reflux and observe the passage of fluid through the pyloric channel (see p. 148).

2. **Position of the patient**. The patient should be lying on his or her back (supine) and may be turned obliquely if necessary. It may be useful to scan the patient erect.

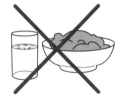

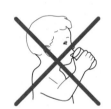

3–4 hours
(except for pyloric stenosis)

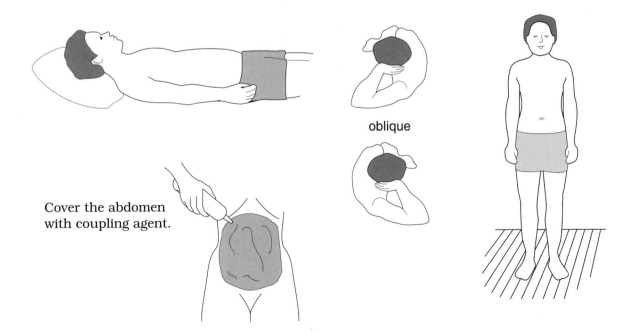

Cover the abdomen with coupling agent.

oblique

3. **Choice of transducer**. For adults, use a 3.5 MHz transducer. For children and thin adults, use a 5 MHz or 7.5 MHz transducer.

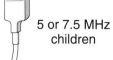

3.5 MHz adults

5 or 7.5 MHz children

4. **Setting the correct gain**. Start by placing the transducer centrally at the top of the abdomen (the xiphoid angle). Angle the beam to the right side of the patient to image the liver; adjust the gain to obtain the best image (see p. 50).

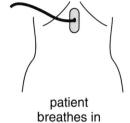

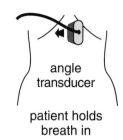

angle transducer

patient breathes in

patient holds breath in

Scanning technique

Start with longitudinal scans, covering the whole abdomen; then add transverse and oblique scans, with pressure if necessary to displace the gas in the bowel.

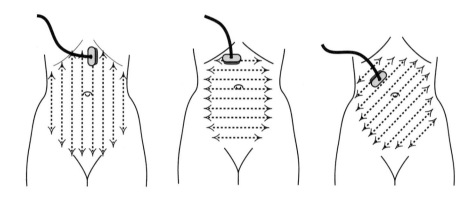

If ascites is suspected, see p. 142.

Correlation with X-rays may be helpful because ultrasound cannot exclude perforation of the bowel. Review antero–posterior supine and erect (or decubitus) projections.

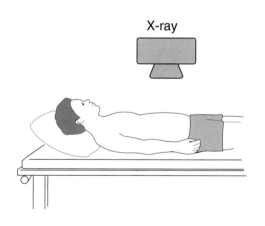

X-ray

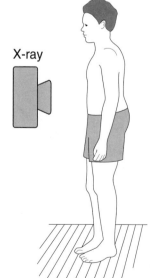

X-ray

Normal gastrointestinal tract

The different anatomical parts of the gastrointestinal tract can be recognized.

The oesophagus

The abdominal part of the oesophagus can be visualized with longitudinal scans, lying inferior to the diaphragm and anterior to the aorta. With transverse scans, the oesophagus is seen behind the left lobe of the liver (Fig. 85).

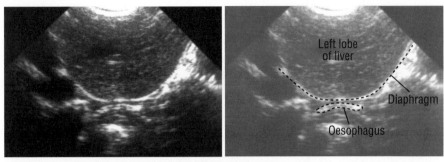

Fig. 85a. Longitudinal scan: the lower oesophagus of a child.

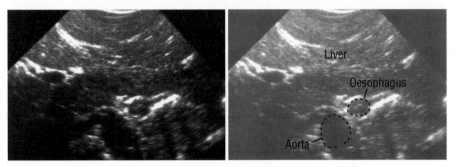

Fig. 85b. Transverse scan: the lower oesophagus of the same child.

The stomach

When empty, the fundus of the stomach will be star-shaped and easily identified (Fig. 86). The body of the stomach will be seen on transverse scanning, just anterior to the pancreas. If there is confusion, give the patient one or two glasses of water to distend the stomach.

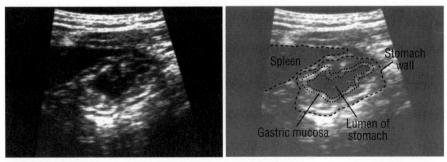

Fig. 86a. Transverse scan: the fundus of a normal stomach.

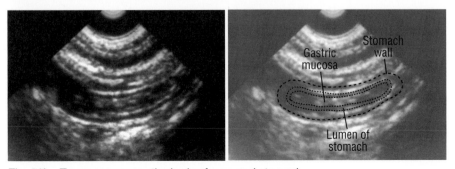

Fig. 86b. Transverse scan: the body of a normal stomach.

Small and large bowel

The appearance of the bowel varies greatly depending upon the degree of fullness, the liquid content and the amount of faeces and gas. Normal peristalsis may be seen on scanning. If the bowel is full of fluid, there will be characteristic mobile echoes. Peristalsis is usually seen in the small bowel but not always in the colon.

With ultrasound, the wall of the intestine is seen as two layers: an external hypoechogenic layer (the muscle) and an internal hyperechogenic layer (the mucosa in contact with gas in the bowel). The muscle wall is seldom more than 3 mm thick, depending on the part of the bowel and the degree of filling (Fig. 87).

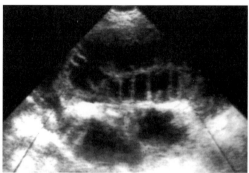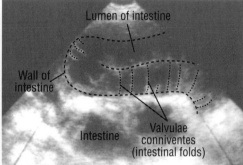

Fig. 87. A fluid-filled loop of small intestine.

The *gas* within the bowel is hyperechogenic and may produce reverberation artefacts and an acoustic shadow posteriorly (Fig. 88), while *fluid* within the bowel is echo-free or may produce some echoes due to faeces.

The normal movements due to respiration should be recognized and differentiated from peristalsis.

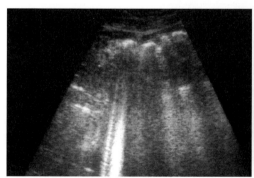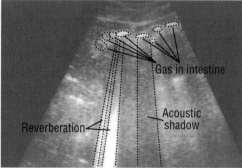

Fig. 88. Reverberation artefacts and an acoustic shadow below gas in the intestine.

Intraperitoneal fluid (ascites)

> **Ultrasound is an accurate way of locating free fluid in the peritoneal cavity.**

The patient should lie on his or her back while the whole abdomen is scanned, and then obliquely on the right or left side as each flank is scanned. If there is excessive gas in the bowel, the hands/knees position can also be used. When searching for fluid, scan the most dependent part of the abdomen in all positions. Fluid will appear as an echo-free area.

Small quantities of fluid will collect in two areas of the abdomen:

1. In women, in the retrouterine cul-de-sac (the pouch of Douglas) (Fig. 89a).

2. In men, in the hepatorenal recess (Morrison's pouch) (Fig. 89b).

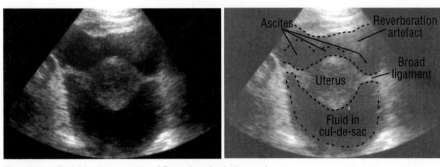

Fig. 89a. Fluid in the pouch of Douglas (cul-de-sac).

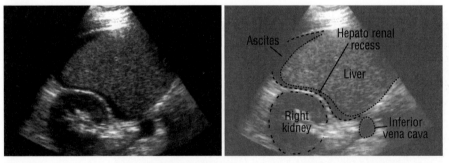

Fig. 89b. Transverse scan: fluid in the hepatorenal recess (Morrison's pouch).

With greater quantities of fluid, the flank spaces (parietocolic gutters) will contain fluid. As the quantity increases, the fluid will fill the whole of the abdominal cavity. The bowel loops will float in the fluid, bringing the intraluminal gas close to the anterior abdominal wall, and will move as the position of the patient changes. If the mesentery is thickened by malignant infiltration or by infection, the bowel will be less free to move and there will be fluid between the abdominal wall and the intestinal loops.

> **Ultrasound cannot distinguish between ascites, blood, bile, pus and urine. Aspiration is necessary to identify the fluid.**

Adhesions in the peritoneal cavity cause septation, and fluid may be obscured by intraluminal or extralumenal gas. Multiple scans in different positions will be required.

Large cysts may simulate ascites. Scan the whole abdomen for fluid, particularly the flanks and pelvis.

> **Ultrasound helps needle aspiration of small quantities of fluid, but training is required (see pp. 318–319).**

Masses in the bowel

1. **Solid masses in the bowel** may be neoplastic, inflammatory (e.g. amoebic) or due to *Ascaris*. Bowel masses are usually kidney-shaped. Ultrasound can show wall thickening, and an irregular, swollen and ill-defined outline (Fig. 90a, b). Infection or spread of a tumour may cause fixation, and associated fluid may be due to perforation or haemorrhage. Localization may be difficult.

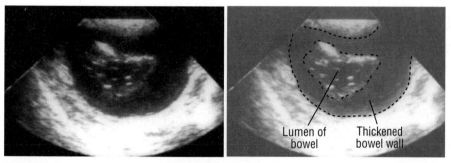

Fig. 90a. Transverse scan: thickened bowel wall.

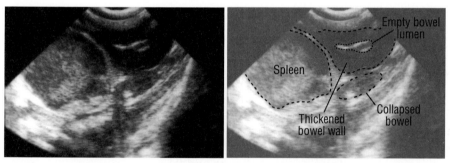

Fig. 90b. Longitudinal scan of the same patient. The thickening of the bowel was due to lymphoma. Most masses in the bowel appear kidney-shaped when imaged by ultrasound.

When a bowel mass is identified, liver metastases must be excluded, as well as enlarged, echo-free mesenteric lymph nodes (Fig. 90c). Normal lymph nodes are seldom seen by ultrasound.

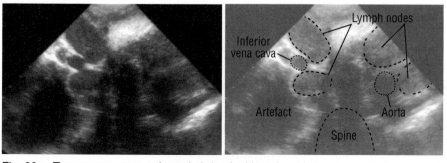

Fig. 90c. Transverse scan: enlarged abdominal lymph nodes.

2. **Solid masses outside the bowel**. Multiple, often confluent and hypoechogenic masses suggest lymphoma or enlarged lymph nodes. In children in the tropics, consider Burkitt lymphoma and scan the kidneys and ovaries for similar tumours. However, the ultrasound differentiation of lymphoma from tuberculous adenitis can be very difficult (Fig. 91).

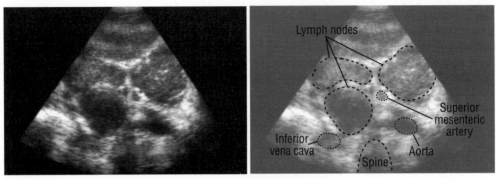

Fig. 91a. Transverse scan: tuberculous lymph nodes. Lymphoma would have a similar appearance.

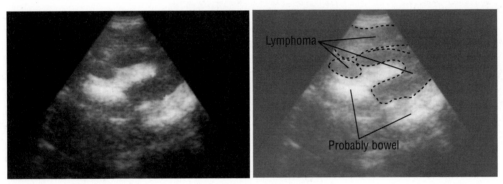

Fig. 91b. Retroperitoneal masses in a child due to lymphoma.

Retroperitoneal sarcoma is uncommon but may present as a large, solid mass of varying echogenicity (see also p. 68). Necrosis may occur centrally, appearing as a hypoechogenic or non-homogeneous area due to liquefaction.

3. **Complex masses**

   • Abscess: may be anywhere in the abdomen or pelvis. It is often tender, with associated fever, poorly outlined and irregular. Apart from appendiceal abscess (see p. 147), consider:

     – colonic diverticulitis with perforation: the abscess is usually in the left lower abdomen;

     – amoebiasis, with perforation: the abscess is usually in the right lower abdomen, less often on the left side or elsewhere;

     – perforation of a neoplasm: the abscess can be anywhere;

     – tuberculosis or other granulomatous infections: the abscess is commonly on the right of the abdomen, but can be anywhere;

     – regional ileitis (Crohn disease), ulcerative colitis, typhoid and other bowel infections: the abscess can be anywhere;

     – perforation by parasites, e.g. *Strongyloides*, *Ascaris* or *Oesophagostomum*: the abscess is usually in the right lower abdomen, but can be anywhere. (*Ascaris* may be identified in cross-section or as long, tubular structures: see p. 149).

It is often easy to identify an abscess, but it is seldom possible to identify the cause.

- A haematoma appears as a cystic or complex mass, similar to an abscess but often apyrexial. A clinical history of recent trauma or anticoagulant therapy is important. Haematomas may show central debris and liquefaction, and may be loculated. Search also for free abdominal fluid (see pp. 142–143).

4. **Fluid-filled masses**. The majority are benign and are either congenital or due to parasitic or other infections. (See pp. 216–217 for gynaecological cysts.)

   - Duplication of the bowel. These congenital lesions often appear as fluid-filled variable shapes with well defined walls. They can be large or small and may contain echoes due to debris or septations (Fig. 92a).

   - Lymphatic or mesenteric cysts. Although usually echo-free, these may be septate, with or without internal echoes. They may be found in any part of the abdominal cavity and are variable in size, up to 20 cm or more in diameter (Fig. 92b).

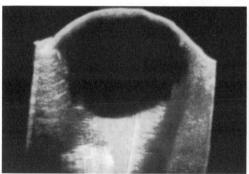 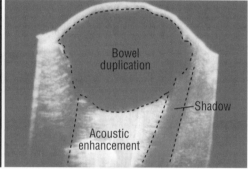

Fig. 92a. Duplication of the bowel.

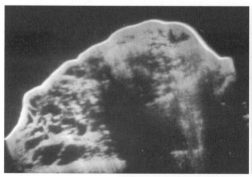 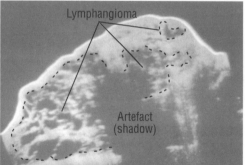

Fig. 92b. An intra-abdominal lymphangioma.

5. **Bowel ischaemia**. Ultrasound will show solid thickening of the bowel wall, sometimes localized but occasionally extensive. Mobile gas bubbles may be found in the portal vein.

6. **Echinococcal cysts (hydatid disease).** Cysts in the abdomen have no specific characteristics and resemble other visceral hydatid cysts, particularly those in the liver. They are almost always multiple, and associated with others elsewhere. (Scan the liver and X-ray the chest.) If there are multiple small clustered cysts, suspect the less common alveolar hydatids *(Echinococcus multilocularis)*.

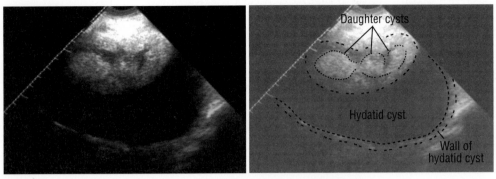

Fig. 93a. A hydatid cyst in the peritoneum with internal daughter cysts.

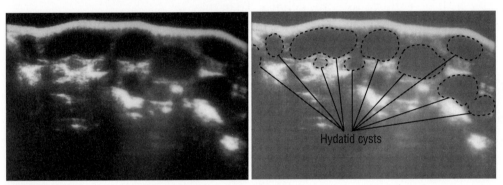

Fig. 93b. Multiple intraperitoneal hydatid cysts.

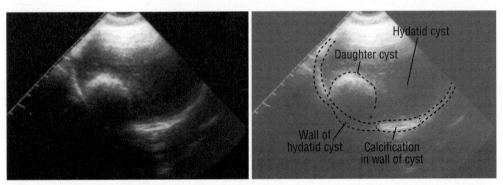

Fig. 93c. A mesenteric hydatid cyst with an internal daughter cyst. There is calcification in the wall of the larger cyst.

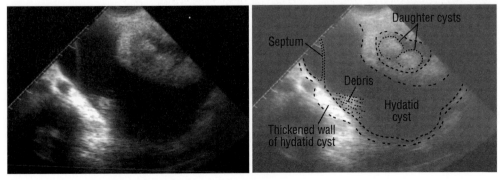

Fig. 93d. A septate intra-abdominal hydatid cyst.

Suspected appendicitis

The diagnosis of acute appendicitis with ultrasound can be difficult and unreliable. Considerable experience is required.

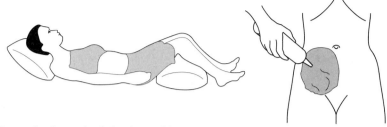

When acute appendicitis is suspected, scan with the patient supine, using a 5 MHz transducer. Put a pillow under both knees to relax the abdomen. Apply coupling agent liberally to the right lower abdomen and start with longitudinal scans, using gentle pressure at first. Use firmer pressure to displace the bowel. If the bowel loops are inflamed, they will be fixed and without peristalsis: tenderness will help localization.

An inflamed appendix appears on cross-sectional scans as fixed, concentric circles (a "target") (Fig. 94a left). The inner lumen will be hypoechogenic, surrounded by hyperechogenic oedema: surrounding the oedema will be hypoechogenic bowel wall. In the long axis, the same pattern will appear in tubular form (Fig. 94a right). If the appendix has perforated, there will be an irregular echo-free or complex area nearby, possibly extending into the pelvis or elsewhere (Fig. 94b).

It is not always easy to demonstrate the appendix, particularly if there is an abscess. Other causes of an abscess in the right lower abdomen include perforation of the bowel due to amoebiasis, neoplasm or parasites (see p. 144). Careful correlation of the ultrasound images with the clinical condition of the patient is essential, but it may not always be possible to make an exact diagnosis with ultrasound.

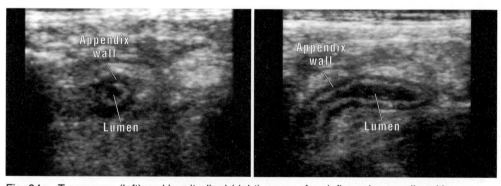

Fig. 94a. Transverse (left) and longitudinal (right) scans of an inflamed appendix, with thickened oedematous walls and surrounding oedema.

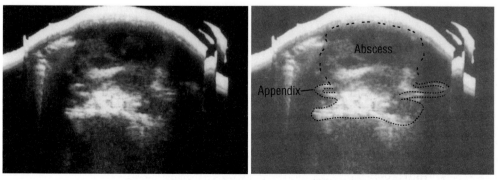

Fig. 94b. Transverse scan: an inflamed, ruptured appendix with resulting abscess.

Gastrointestinal symptoms in children

Ultrasound is particularly useful in the following paediatric conditions.

Hypertrophic pyloric stenosis

The diagnosis will be made clinically in the majority of infants by palpating the olive-shaped thickening of the pylorus. This can easily be shown by ultrasound and accurately diagnosed (Fig. 95). There will be a hypoechogenic region due to the thickened pyloric muscle, which should normally not exceed 4 mm. The transverse internal diameter of the pyloric canal should not exceed 2 mm. Gastric stasis will be demonstrated even before giving the infant the warm, sweet drink which is necessary to fill the stomach before the rest of the examination (see p. 138).

In longitudinal scans, the length of the pyloric canal in infancy should not exceed 2 cm. Any measurement in excess of this strongly suggests hypertrophic pyloric stenosis.

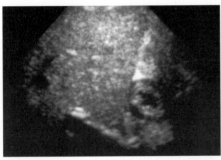
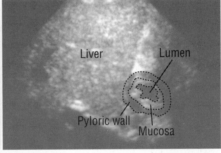

Fig. 95a. Transverse scan: a normal infant pylorus.

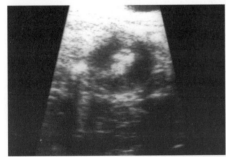
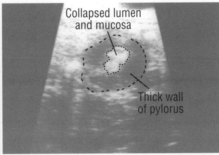

Fig. 95b. Transverse scan: infantile pyloric hypertrophy.

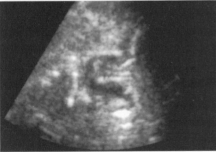
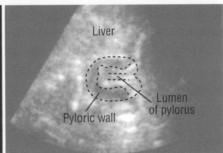

Fig. 95c. Longitudinal scan: normal infant pylorus.

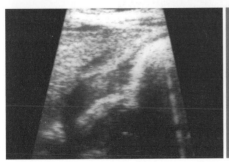
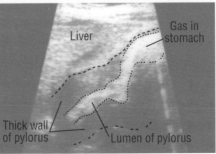

Fig. 95d. Longitudinal scan: infantile pyloric hypertrophy.

Intussusception

When clinical examination suggests intussusception, scanning the abdomen will sometimes demonstrate the characteristic sausage-shaped invagination: if seen in transverse sections, the concentric rings of bowel are also characteristic (Fig. 96a). There will be a peripheral rim which is hypoechogenic, at least 8 mm thick and with an overall diameter of more than 3 cm.

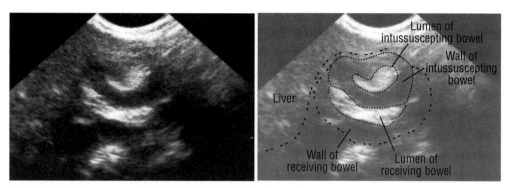

Fig. 96a. Transverse scan: intussusception of the bowel.

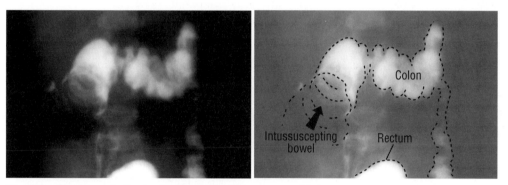

Fig. 96b. Radiograph: the barium enema of the same patient.

In children, the ultrasound diagnosis of hypertrophic pyloric stenosis and intussusception needs experience and close clinical correlation.

Ascaris

Masses in any part of the bowel may be due to *Ascaris*: the typical concentric rings of the bowel wall and the body of the contained worm may be seen when scanned in transverse section. *Ascaris* will probably be mobile and movement may be observed in real-time scanning. Perforation into the peritoneal cavity may occur.

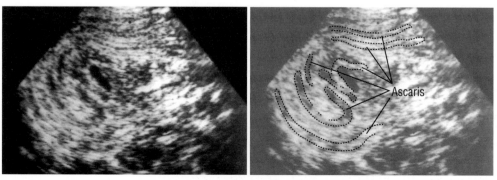

Fig. 96c. Numerous *Ascaris* (roundworms) in the small intestine of a child.

Infection with human immunodeficiency virus

HIV-infected patients are often pyrexial, but the source of the infection cannot always be identified by clinical examination. Ultrasound is helpful in localizing abdominal abscesses or enlarged lymph nodes. When there is intestinal obstruction, the dilated small bowel, with an abnormal mucosal pattern, may be recognized early with ultrasound.

Following standard techniques, the ultrasound examination should always include:

1. The liver.
2. The spleen.
3. Both subphrenic regions.
4. The kidneys.
5. The pelvis.
6. Any localized subcutaneous swelling or tenderness.
7. The para-aortic and pelvic lymph nodes.

Ultrasound cannot differentiate between bacterial and fungal infections. If an abscess contains gas, it is likely to be a predominantly bacterial infection, although mixed bacterial and fungal abscesses may occur.

> **When a patient who is HIV-positive becomes pyrexial, abdominal and pelvic ultrasound examination is recommended.**

CHAPTER 13
Kidneys and ureters

Indications

1. Renal or ureteric pain.
2. Suspected renal mass (large kidney).
3. Non-functioning kidney on urography.
4. Haematuria.
5. Recurrent urinary infection.
6. Trauma.
7. Suspected polycystic disease.
8. Pyrexia of unknown origin or postoperative complication.
9. Renal failure of unknown origin.
10. Schistosomiasis.

Ultrasound *cannot* assess renal function.

Preparation

1. **Preparation of the patient**. No preparation is required. If the urinary bladder is to be examined, the patient should drink water (see p. 176).

2. **Position of the patient**. Start with the patient lying on his/her back (supine).

   Cover the right upper abdomen liberally with coupling agent.

3. **Choice of transducer**. For adults, use a 3.5 MHz transducer. For children and thin adults, use a 5.0 MHz transducer.

4. **Setting the correct gain**. Start by placing the transducer over the right upper abdomen. Angle the beam as necessary and adjust the gain to obtain the best image of the renal parenchyma.

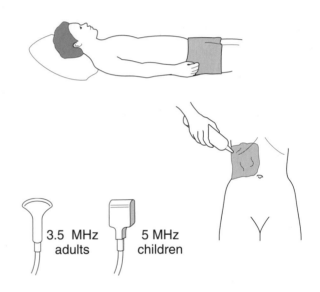

3.5 MHz adults   5 MHz children

Scanning technique

The right kidney can be seen best with the patient supine, using the liver as an acoustic window.

Scanning is always done in deep suspended inspiration: ask the patient to take a deep breath and hold the breath in. Do not forget to tell the patient to relax and breathe normally again.

Start with a longitudinal scan over the right upper abdomen and then follow with a transverse scan. Next, rotate the patient to the left lateral decubitus position, to visualize the right kidney in this coronal view.

Patient holds breath in during scanning.

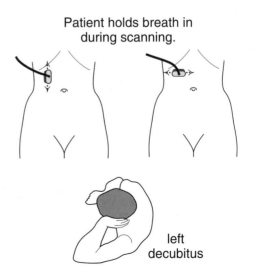

left decubitus

To visualize the left kidney, apply coupling agent to the left upper abdomen. Scan the left kidney in a similar sequence.

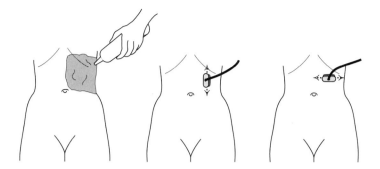

If the left kidney cannot be seen (usually because of excess bowel gas), try the right decubitus position (lying on the right side).

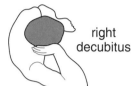

right decubitus

Bowel gas can also be displaced if the patient drinks 3 or 4 glasses of water. The left kidney can then be visualized through the fluid-filled stomach with the patient in the supine position.

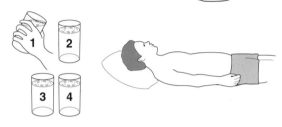

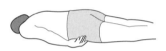

If the kidneys have not been imaged adequately, scan through the lower intercostal spaces. Turn the patient prone and apply coupling agent to the left and right renal area. Perform longitudinal and transverse scans over both renal areas.

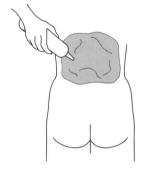
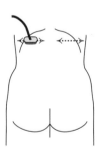
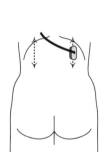
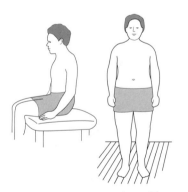

Both kidneys can also be examined with the patient sitting or standing erect.

erect position useful for large patients

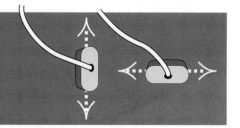

Whatever position is used, remember to scan the kidneys in both longitudinal and transverse planes.

When examining any part of the renal area, compare both kidneys in different projections. Variations in size, contour and internal echogenicity may indicate an abnormality.

Normal kidney

Measurements made with ultrasound are generally less than those made by radiography; they are more accurate.

Both kidneys should be about the same size. In adults, a difference of more than 2 cm in length is abnormal.

1. Length: up to 12 cm and not less than 9 cm

   length: more than 9 cm, less than 12 cm

2. Width: normally 4–6 cm but may vary a little with the angle of the scan

   width: between 4 cm and 6 cm (varies with angle of scan)

3. Thickness: up to 3.5 cm but may vary a little with the angle of the scan

   thickness: less than 3.5 cm (varies with angle of scan)

4. The central echo complex (the renal sinus) is very echogenic and normally occupies about one-third of the kidney (Fig. 97). (The renal sinus includes the pelvis, calyces, vessels and fat.)

   renal sinus: usually about 1/3 of the kidney

In the newborn, the kidneys are about 4 cm long and 2 cm wide (see p. 287 for growth progress).

The renal pyramids are poorly defined hypoechogenic areas in the medulla of the kidney, surrounded by the more echogenic renal cortex. It is easier to see the pyramids in children and young adults.

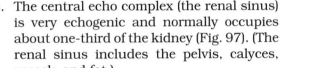

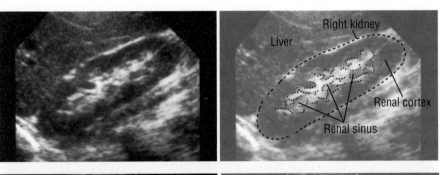

Fig. 97a. Longitudinal scan of a normal right kidney.

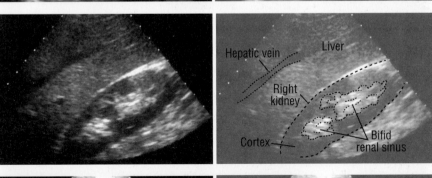

Fig. 97b. Longitudinal scan of a normal right kidney with a bifid renal sinus.

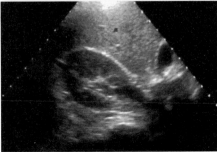

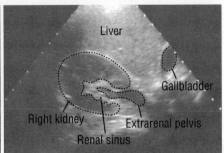

Fig. 97c. Anterior transverse scan through the right renal sinus, showing the pelvis.

When scanning it is important to identify the following:

1. The renal capsule. This appears as a bright, smooth, echogenic line around the kidney.

2. The cortex. This is less echogenic than the liver but more echogenic than the adjacent renal pyramids (Fig. 98a).

3. The renal medulla. This contains the hypoechogenic, renal pyramids which should not be mistaken for renal cysts.

4. The renal sinus (the fat, the collecting system and the vessels at the hilus). This is the innermost part of the kidney and has the greatest echogenicity (Fig. 98b).

5. The ureters. Normal ureters are not always seen: they should be sought where they leave the kidney at the hilus (Fig. 98c). They may be single or multiple and are often seen in the coronal projection.

6. The renal arteries and veins. These are best seen at the hilus. They may be multiple and may enter the kidney at different levels (Fig. 98c).

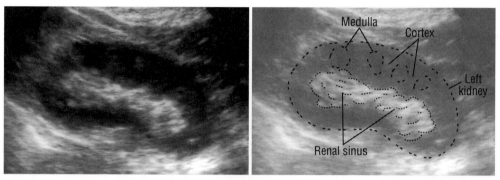

Fig. 98a. Longitudinal scan of a normal left kidney.

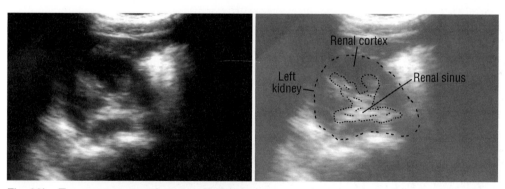

Fig. 98b. Transverse scan of a normal left kidney.

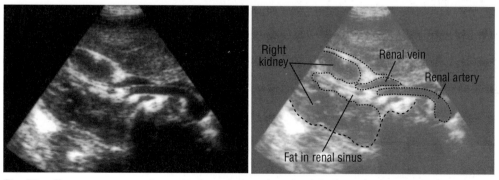

Fig. 98c. Transverse scan of a normal renal sinus (renal pelvis, fat and vessels).

Adrenal (suprarenal) glands

The adrenal glands are not easily seen with ultrasound. The best scanning positions are with the patient supine, imaging as for the inferior vena cava, and with the patient in the lateral decubitus position (coronal scan). The adrenals are situated above and medial to the kidneys. If they are easy to see, they are likely to be pathologically enlarged, except in infants (Fig. 99).

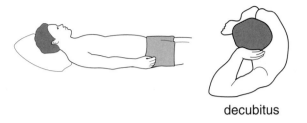

decubitus

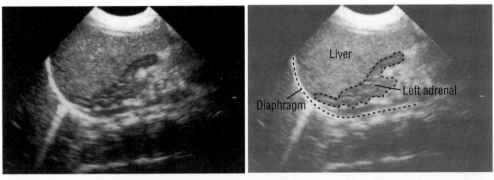

Fig. 99a. Longitudinal scan of the normal left adrenal gland of an infant (the adrenals are large compared with those of an adult).

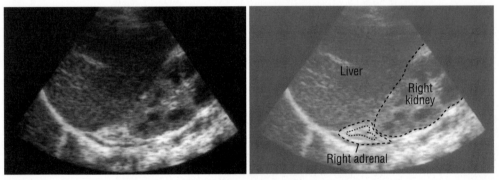

Fig. 99b. Longitudinal scan of a normal right adrenal gland of an adult.

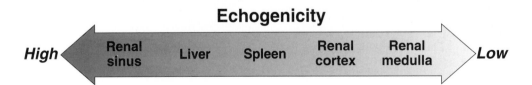

Warning: renal pyramids may be confused with renal cysts or tumours. Adjust the gain settings.

Echogenicity

High — Renal sinus — Liver — Spleen — Renal cortex — Renal medulla — Low

Absent kidney

If either kidney cannot be seen, search again. Adjust the gain to show the liver parenchyma and spleen, and scan in different projections. Assess the size of the visible kidney. Hypertrophy of a kidney occurs (at any age) in a few months when the other kidney has been removed or is not functioning. If there is one large kidney and the other cannot be visualized after a careful search, it is probable that the patient has only one kidney.

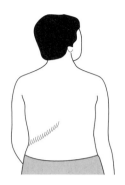

If one kidney cannot be demonstrated, consider the following possibilities:

1. The kidney may have been removed. Check the clinical history and examine the patient for scars.

2. The kidney may be ectopic. Search the kidney area and the whole abdomen, including the pelvis (Fig. 100). If no kidney is found, X-ray the chest. A contrast urogram may be necessary.

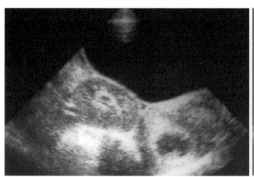
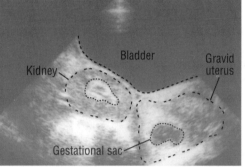

Fig. 100. Longitudinal scan through the bladder showing a low-lying (pelvic) kidney. The patient is 8 weeks pregnant.

> **A pelvic kidney may be confused sonographically with a tubo-ovarian mass or gastrointestinal tumour. Use a contrast urogram to locate the kidney.**

3. If only one large but normal kidney is demonstrated, and there has not been any surgery, it is likely that there is congenital absence of the other kidney. If the only kidney visualized is not enlarged, a failure to demonstrate the other kidney suggests chronic disease.

4. If there is one large but distorted kidney, there may be a developmental abnormality.

5. Apparent absence of both kidneys may be a failure to demonstrate them with ultrasound because of changed echogenicity resulting from chronic disease of the renal parenchyma.

6. Any kidney less than 2 cm thick and 4 cm long can be very difficult to visualize. Locate a renal vessel or ureter; this may help to localize the kidney, especially if the ureter is dilated.

Large kidney

Bilateral enlargement

1. When the kidneys are enlarged but normal in shape, with normal, decreased or increased homogeneous echogenicity, the possible causes are:

   - Acute or subacute glomerulonephritis or severe pyelonephritis (Fig. 101a).

   - Amyloidosis (probably increased echogenicity) (Fig. 101b).

   - The nephrotic syndrome.

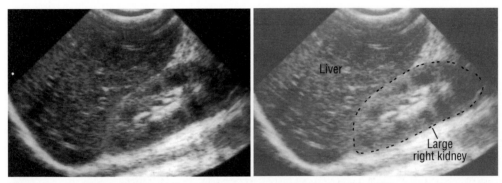

Fig. 101a. Longitudinal scan: a large kidney due to glomerulonephritis. (Size must always be confirmed by measurement.)

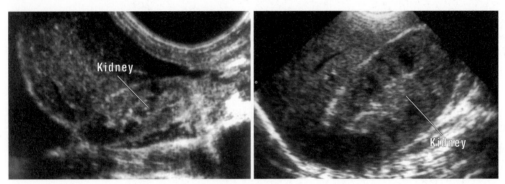

Fig. 101b. Two longitudinal scans: enlarged hyperechogenic kidneys in two patients with amyloidosis. The differentiation between renal cortex and sinus is no longer so clearly visible.

2. When the kidneys have a smooth outline and are uniformly enlarged, with non-homogeneous hyperechogenicity, the possible causes are:

   - Lymphoma. This may cause multiple areas of low density, especially Burkitt lymphoma in children or young adults (Fig. 102).

   - Metastases (Fig. 102).

   - Polycystic kidneys (see p. 162).

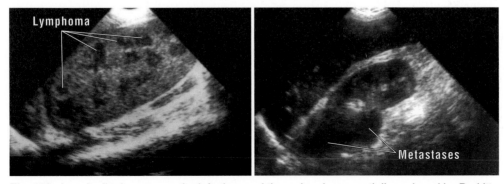

Fig. 102. Longitudinal scans: on the left, the renal tissue has been partially replaced by Burkitt lymphoma; on the right, by metastases.

Unilateral enlargement

If one kidney appears to be enlarged but has normal echogenicity, and the other kidney is small or absent, the enlargement may be due to compensatory hypertrophy. When no other kidney is seen, exclude crossed ectopia and other developmental abnormality (Fig. 103a, b).

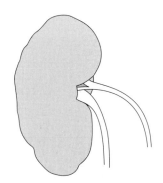

The kidney may be slightly enlarged because of persistent segmentation (duplication) with two or even three ureters. Search for the renal hilus: there are likely to be two or more vessels and ureters. A contrast urogram may be necessary.

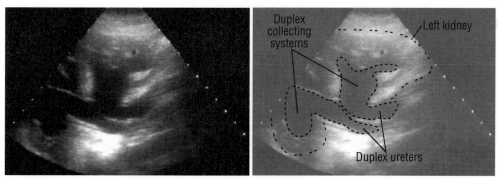

Fig. 103a. Longitudinal scan: an unobstructed duplex kidney.

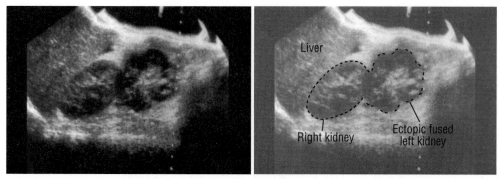

Fig. 103b. Longitudinal posterior scan: an obstructed (hydronephrotic) duplex left kidney.

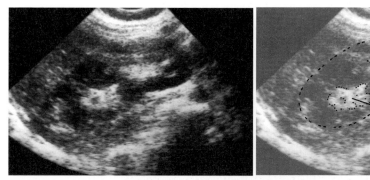

Fig. 103c. Transverse scan: crossed fused renal ectopia.

One kidney is enlarged or more lobulated than normal

The commonest cause of an enlarged kidney is hydronephrosis, which will appear on ultrasound images as multiple, well circumscribed cystic areas (the calyces) with a dilated central cystic area (the renal pelvis, normally less than 1 cm in width). Coronal images will show the continuity between the calyces and the pelvis. In multicystic kidneys there is no such continuity (see p. 162).

Degrees of hydronephrosis

Normal

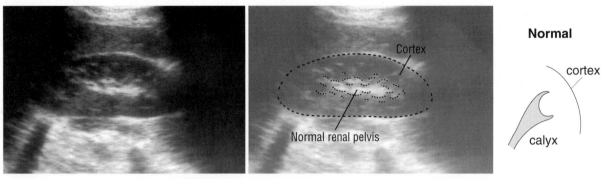

Fig. 104a. Longitudinal scan: the renal pelvis of a normal kidney is less than 1 cm in width.

Mild

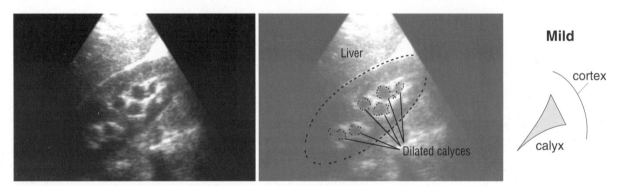

Fig. 104b. Longitudinal scan: a renal pelvis more than 1 cm in width, indicating mild hydronephrosis. Small parapelvic cysts have a similar appearance.

Moderate

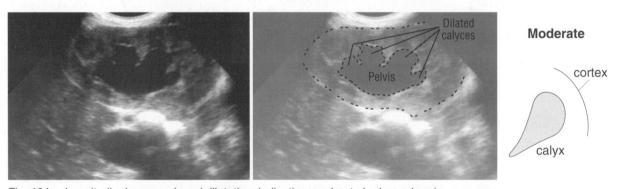

Fig. 104c. Longitudinal scan: calyceal dilatation, indicating moderate hydronephrosis.

Severe

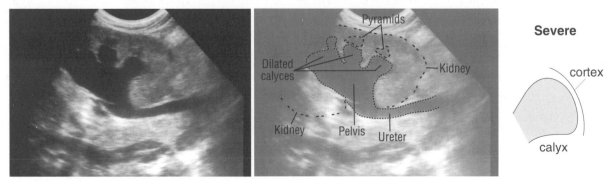

Fig. 104d. Longitudinal scan: dilated calyces and a renal cortex decreased in width are indicative of advanced hydronephrosis.

Always compare the two kidneys when assessing the size of the renal pelvis. When much of the pelvis is outside the renal parenchyma, it may be a normal variant. When the renal pelvis is enlarged, normal echoes can be lost because of the fluid content (Fig. 105a).

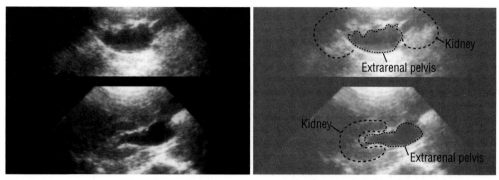

Fig. 105a. Longitudinal (upper) and transverse (lower) scans: a kidney with a large extrarenal pelvis.

A large renal pelvis may be due either to overhydration with increased urinary output or to an overfilled urinary bladder. The renal calyces will be normal. Ask the patient to empty the bladder and rescan (Fig. 105b).

Pelvic dilatation can occur normally in pregnancy and does not necessarily indicate infection. Check the urine for infection, and check the uterus for pregnancy.

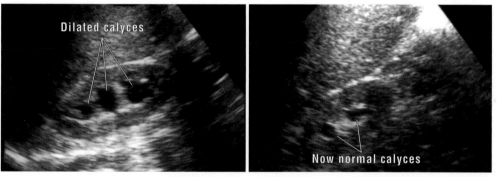

Fig. 105b. Dilated calyces due to overhydration (left) which become normal after micturition (right).

A large renal pelvis is an indication to scan the ureters and the bladder and particularly the other kidney to locate the obstruction. If no cause is identified, a contrast urogram will be necessary. The normal convex calyces may become inverted and rounded as the degree of obstruction increases. Eventually the renal cortex becomes thinned (see p. 160).

To assess the degree of hydronephrosis, measure the size of the renal pelvis when the bladder is empty. If the pelvis is wider than 1 cm, but there is no calyceal dilatation, the hydronephrosis is mild. When there is calyceal dilatation, the hydronephrosis is moderate. If there is loss of the renal cortex, it is advanced (Fig. 104).

Hydronephrosis can be caused by congenital obstruction of the uretero-pelvic junction, by ureteric stenosis (e.g. as in schistosomiasis (Fig. 122c, p. 179)) or a calculus, or from external pressure on the ureters by a retroperitoneal or abdominal mass.

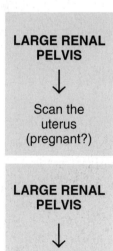

LARGE RENAL PELVIS

↓

Scan the uterus (pregnant?)

LARGE RENAL PELVIS

↓

Scan ureters, bladder, other kidney

Renal cysts

When ultrasound shows multiple, echo-free, well circumscribed areas throughout the kidney, suspect multicystic kidney. This condition is usually unilateral, whereas congenital polycystic kidney disease is almost always bilateral (although the cysts may not be symmetrical) (Fig. 106a).

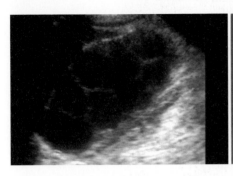
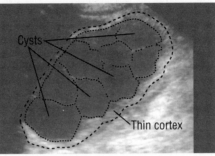

Fig. 106a. Longitudinal scan: multicystic right kidney. All the cysts are approximately the same size.

	Internal echoes	Back wall	Contour	Shape
Cyst	No	Strong	Well defined	Spherical
Tumour	Yes	No change or strong	Irregular	Variable Ill defined

1. Simple cysts can be single or multiple. On ultrasound the walls are smooth and rounded without internal echoes, but with a clearly defined back wall (Fig. 106b, c). Such cysts are usually unilocular and, when multiple, will differ in size. Rarely, these cysts become infected or haemorrhage, producing internal echoes. When this occurs or when the outline of any cyst is irregular, further investigation is required.

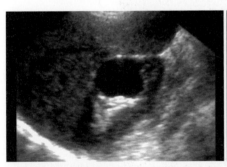
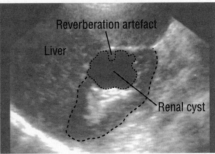

Fig. 106b. Longitudinal scan: a large single cyst in the right kidney.

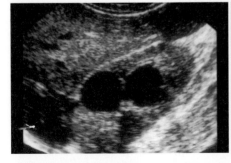
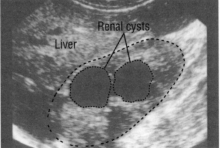

Fig. 106c. Longitudinal scan: multiple renal cysts.

More than 70% of all renal cysts are due to benign cystic disease. These cysts are very common over the age of 50 years and may be bilateral. They seldom cause symptoms.

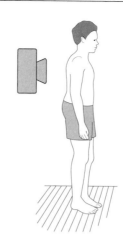

2. Hydatid cysts usually contain debris and are often loculated or septate (Fig. 107a, b). When calcified, the wall appears as a bright, echogenic convex line with acoustic shadowing (Fig. 107c). Hydatid cysts may be multiple or bilateral. Scan the liver for other cysts and X-ray the chest.

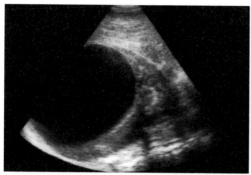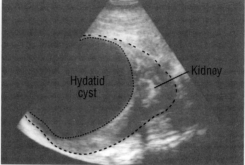

Fig. 107a. Longitudinal scan: a hydatid cyst in a right kidney.

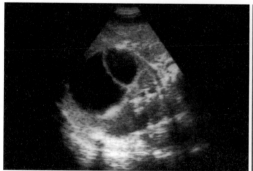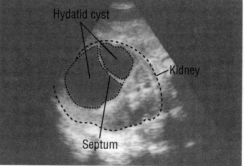

Fig. 107b. Transverse scan: a septate hydatid cyst in a right kidney.

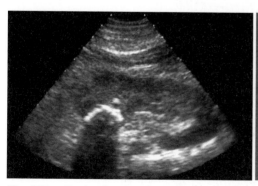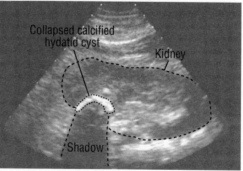

Fig. 107c. Supine longitudinal scan: a collapsed calcified hydatid cyst in the upper pole of a left kidney.

3. If there are multiple cysts in one kidney, the kidney is usually enlarged. This may indicate alveolar echinococcosis. If the patient is less than 50 years old and clinically well, check the other kidney to exclude polycystic disease: congenital cysts are echo-free and without mural calcification. Both kidneys are always enlarged (see p. 162).

Renal masses

> **Ultrasound cannot reliably differentiate between benign renal tumours (other than renal cysts) and malignant renal tumours, and cannot always accurately differentiate malignant tumours from renal abscesses.**

There are two exceptions to the above statement:

1. In the early stages, a renal angiomyolipoma (Fig. 108a) has ultrasound characteristics that allow accurate recognition. These tumours can occur at any age and may be bilateral. Ultrasound images show a well circumscribed, hyperechogenic and homogeneous mass, and as the tumour grows there will be back wall attenuation. However, some tumours will undergo central necrosis and there will be strong back wall echoes. At this stage differentiation by ultrasound is no longer possible, but abdominal X-rays may show fat within the tumour, which is unlikely to occur in any other type of renal mass.

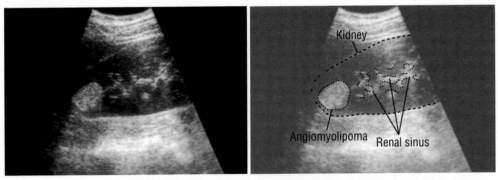

Fig. 108a. Supine longitudinal scan: an angiomyolipoma in a right kidney.

2. When a renal tumour spreads into the inferior vena cava or into the perirenal tissues, there is no doubt that the tumour is malignant (Fig. 108b). (See also p. 166.)

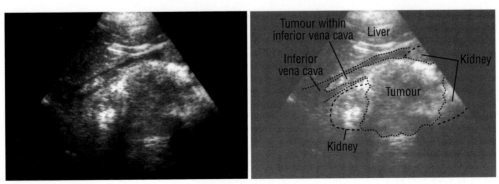

Fig. 108b. Longitudinal scan: a large renal tumour involving the inferior vena cava and spreading beyond the renal capsule.

Solid renal mass

Renal masses may be well circumscribed or irregular and may alter the shape of the kidney. Echogenicity may be increased or decreased. In the early stages, the majority of malignant tumours are homogeneous: if central necrosis occurs, they become non-homogeneous (Fig.109a, b, c).

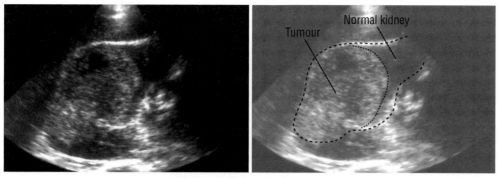

Fig. 109a. Oblique longitudinal scan: a well-circumscribed tumour in a right kidney.

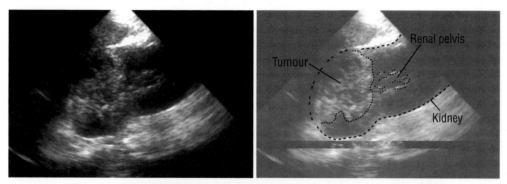

Fig. 109b. Oblique longitudinal scan: an irregular, ill-defined tumour in a right kidney.

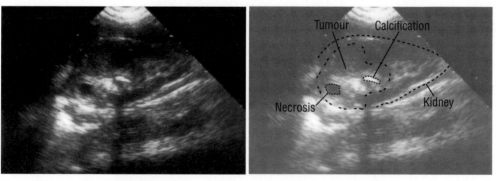

Fig. 109c. Longitudinal scan: a tumour with central necrosis in a right kidney.

It is important to recognize normal or hypertrophied columns of Bertin, which can resemble a tumour (Fig. 110). The echo pattern of the cortex should be the same as the rest of the kidney; however, in some patients, differentiation may be difficult.

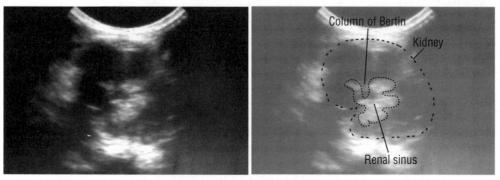

Fig. 110. Transverse scan: a normal prominent column of Bertin.

A complex non-homogeneous mass

The differential diagnosis of complex masses can be very difficult, but when there is spread of a tumour beyond the kidney, there is no doubt that it is malignant (Fig. 111a, b). Malignant tumours may also be contained within the kidney (see p. 165). Both tumours and haematomas may show acoustic shadowing due to calcification.

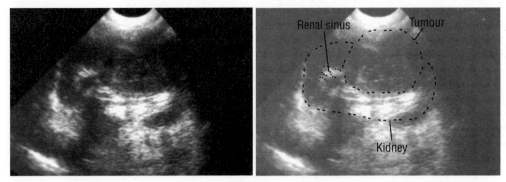

Fig. 111a. Longitudinal scan: a tumour in a left kidney, which is invading the renal tissue and beyond it (renal carcinoma).

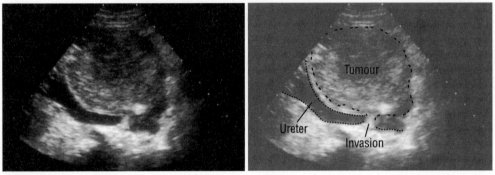

Fig. 111b. Transverse scan: a tumour in the lower pole of a left kidney, invading the left ureter and causing obstructive hydronephrosis.

As a tumour grows, its centre may become necrotic with a rough irregular outline and much internal debris, causing a complex ultrasound pattern. The differentiation of this from an abscess or a haematoma can be difficult. The clinical condition of the patient may indicate the correct diagnosis. Tumours can spread into the renal vein or inferior vena cava and resemble thrombosis (Fig. 111c) (see p. 69).

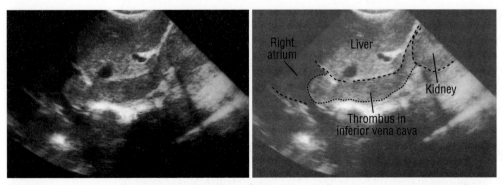

Fig. 111c. Longitudinal scan: a renal tumour invading the renal vein and inferior vena cava, resulting in thrombosis.

Always scan both kidneys. When a malignant renal tumour is suspected (at any age), scan the liver and the inferior vena cava. Also X-ray the chest for metastases.

A rough, irregular, echogenic mass containing debris within an enlarged kidney may be malignant or a pyogenic or tuberculous abscess (Fig. 112a, b, c). The patient's clinical condition may help to differentiate (see also p. 166).

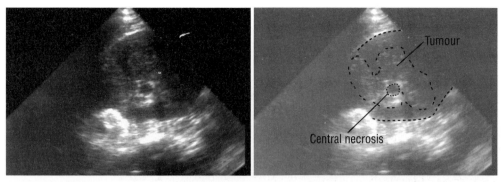

Fig. 112a. Transverse scan: a centrally necrotic renal tumour with internal debris.

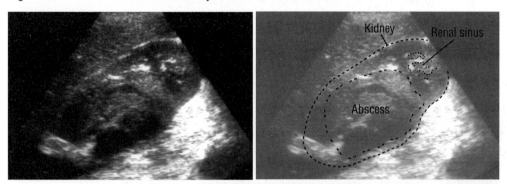

Fig. 112b. Longitudinal scan: a large pyogenic abscess, seen as a complex mass in the right kidney.

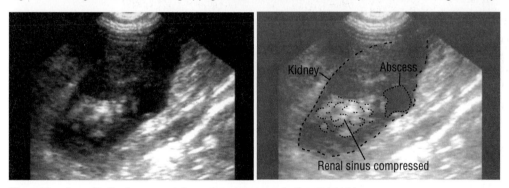

Fig. 112c. Longitudinal scan: a tuberculous abscess in the right kidney.

In children, malignant tumours, e.g. nephroblastoma (Wilms tumour), may be well encapsulated but not homogeneous. Some show calcification but not in the capsule. Haemorrhage or necrosis may change the echogenicity (Fig. 112d). Some are bilateral.

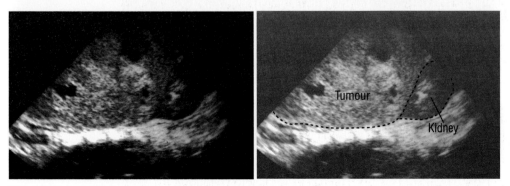

Fig. 112d. Longitudinal scan: a Wilms tumour in the right kidney of a child showing nodularity and areas of necrosis.

Small kidney

1. A small kidney with normal echogenicity may be due to renal artery stenosis or occlusion, or to congenital hypoplasia (Fig. 113a).

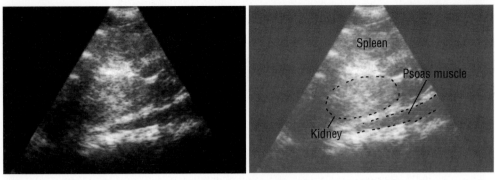

Fig. 113a. Longitudinal scan: a small, isodense but otherwise normal left kidney: the result of renal artery stenosis.

2. A small kidney, normal in shape but hyperechogenic, may indicate chronic renal disease (Fig. 113b). In renal failure, both kidneys are likely to be equally affected.

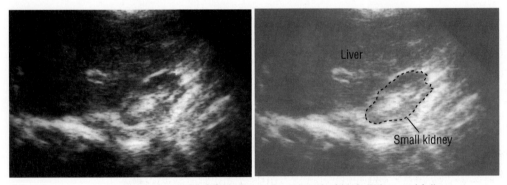

Fig. 113b. Longitudinal scan: a small right kidney, associated with chronic renal failure.

3. A small, hyperechogenic kidney with an irregular, rather "rough" outline and variable thickness of the cortex (usually bilateral but often very asymmetrical) is probably the result of chronic pyelonephritis or infection such as tuberculosis. There may be calcification in the abscesses, showing as bright areas (Fig. 113c).

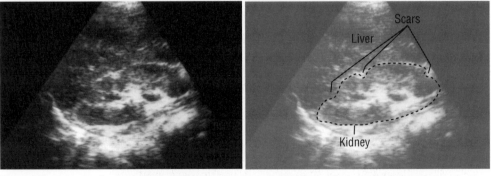

Fig. 113c. Longitudinal scan: a small, irregular (scarred) kidney, the result of chronic pyelonephritis.

4. A single, small, normally shaped but hyperechogenic kidney may be due to end-stage renal vein thrombosis. Acute renal vein thrombosis usually causes renal enlargement, with shrinkage occurring later. Chronic obstructive nephropathy can affect one kidney in the same way, but chronic glomerulonephritis is usually bilateral.

Renal calculi (stones)

Not all calculi can be seen on a plain radiograph of the abdomen, and not all renal calculi can be detected by ultrasound. If clinical symptoms suggest calculi, all patients with a negative ultrasound examination need intravenous contrast urography.

Suspected urinary calculi, urine abnormal but negative ultrasound = intravenous urography.

Calculi are most easily seen in the renal collecting system. The minimum detectable size on a general purpose ultrasound unit, using a 3.5 MHz transducer, is 3–4 mm diameter. Smaller stones (2–3 mm) may be seen with a 5 MHz transducer. A calculus will be hyperechogenic with an acoustic shadow (Fig. 114). The calculus must be visualized in two different planes, longitudinal and transverse, to permit accurate localization and measurement. This may avoid confusion with calcification in the renal parenchyma and other tissues, e.g. the neck of a calyx, which can simulate calculus and give a similar echo and shadow.

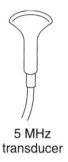

5 MHz
transducer

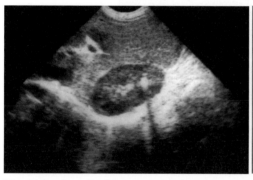 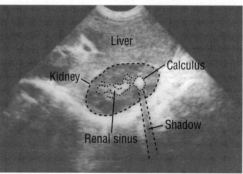

Fig. 114a. Longitudinal scan: a calculus in a right kidney.

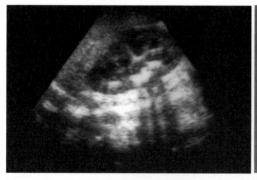 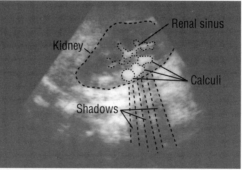

Fig. 114b. Longitudinal scan: multiple calculi in a right kidney.

Ureteric calculi are *very* difficult to locate by ultrasound. *Failure to see a ureteric calculus does not mean that there is no calculus.*

Trauma

1. In the acute stage, renal ultrasound may show intrarenal or perirenal echo-free areas as a result of the presence of blood (haematoma) or extravasated urine (Fig. 115a, b).

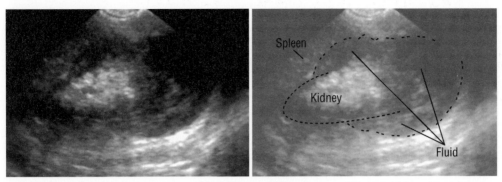

Fig. 115a. Longitudinal scan of an injured patient: the lower pole of the left kidney has been ruptured and there is fluid (blood or urine) around the left kidney.

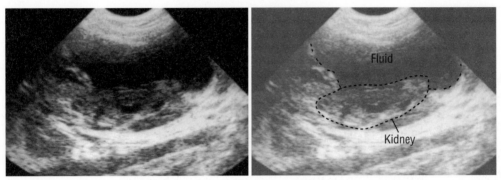

Fig. 115b. Longitudinal scan: fluid around the kidney following injury.

2. When the blood has clotted and formed a thrombus, the same areas will show as bright echoes or a mixture of echo and echo-free areas (a complex mass or masses) (Fig. 115c). In all cases of trauma, check the opposite kidney, but remember that ultrasound cannot assess renal function.

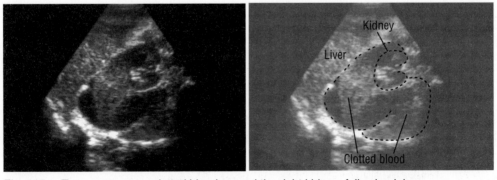

Fig. 115c. Transverse scan: clotted blood around the right kidney, following injury.

Ability to visualize the kidney does *not* mean that it is functioning. To assess renal function, use contrast urography, a radionuclide study or laboratory tests. Remember that injury to a kidney may result in temporary loss of function.

Perirenal fluid

Blood, pus and urine around the kidney cannot be distinguished on ultrasound. All appear as an echo-free area (Fig. 116) (see also p. 170).

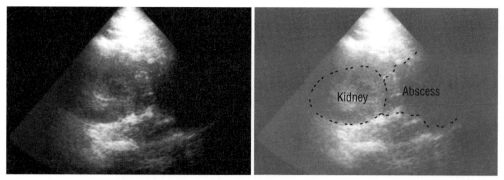

Fig. 116. Transverse scan: a left perirenal abscess.

Retroperitoneal masses

Lymphoma usually presents as a hypoechogenic para-aortic or aorto-caval mass. If the gain is set too low, it may resemble fluid. Any such mass can displace the kidney.

A psoas abscess or haematoma can be echo-free or complex: clotted blood will be hyperechogenic. If there is gas, some areas may be hyperechogenic with acoustic shadows (Fig. 117).

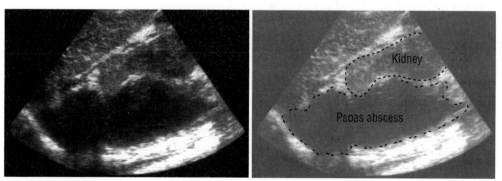

Fig. 117. A large retroperitoneal (psoas) abscess.

Suprarenal mass

Scan both adrenals. A suprarenal mass may be a primary or metastatic tumour, abscess or haematoma. Most are well defined but may become complex. Adrenal haemorrhage is common in the newborn (Fig. 118).

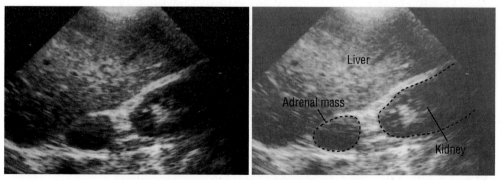

Fig. 118. Longitudinal scan: benign adenoma of the right adrenal gland.

Failure to see an adrenal gland does not exclude abnormality.

Ureters

Because of their position behind the bowel, it is not easy to examine normal ureters by ultrasound. If dilated (e.g. by outlet obstruction due to an enlarged prostate or urethral stricture, or due to vesico-ureteric reflux), they are easier to see, particularly near the kidney or bladder. The middle of the ureters is never seen easily and is much better demonstrated by intravenous urography. However, if thickened, as in schistosomiasis (sometimes with calcification), they can be recognized with ultrasound (Fig. 119) (see also p. 179).

The lower end of the ureters can be observed by scanning through a full bladder, which provides a useful acoustic window.

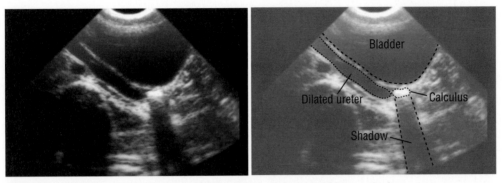

Fig. 119a. Dilatation of the lower end of the right ureter, caused by a calculus.

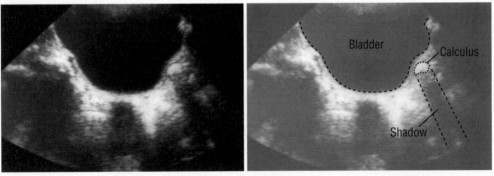

Fig. 119b. Transverse scan: a large calculus at the lower end of the ureter. Small ureteric calculi may be difficult to localize with ultrasound scanning.

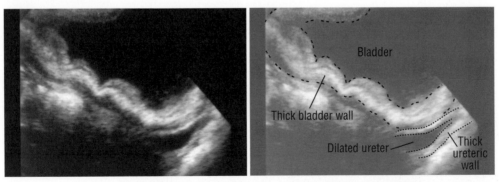

Fig. 119c. Longitudinal scan through the full bladder, showing thickening and dilatation of the lower end of the ureter in a child with schistosomiasis. (Ultrasound scanning is a useful way to monitor treatment of this infection and to differentiate calcification from artefacts.)

Ultrasound is not a reliable way to recognize either ureteric calculi or stenosis.

Renal differential diagnosis

A single large cyst
- Exclude gross hydronephrosis.

Irregular renal outline (not lobulated)
- Consider chronic pyelonephritis or multiple renal infarcts.

Irregular renal outline (smooth)
- Normal lobulation or cystic disease (congenital or parasitic).

Missing kidney
- Ectopia or displacement.
- Surgery.
- Too small to see on ultrasound.
- Replacement by tumour.

Large kidney (normal shape)
- Hydronephrosis.
- Cystic disease.
- Acute renal vein thrombosis.
- Compensatory hypertrophy (other kidney absent or diseased).

Large kidney (asymmetrical shape)
- Tumour.
- Abscess.
- Hydatid cyst.
- Adult polycystic disease.

Small kidney
- Glomerulonephritis.
- Chronic pyelonephritis.
- Infarction or chronic renal vein thrombosis.
- Congenital hypoplasia.

Perirenal fluid*
- Blood.
- Pus.
- Urine.

*Ultrasound cannot distinguish the type of fluid.

Missing kidney? Always check the opposite kidney and in the pelvis.

Notes

CHAPTER 14

Urinary bladder

Indications

1. Dysuria or frequency of micturition.
2. Haematuria (wait until bleeding has stopped).
3. Recurrent infection (cystitis) in adults; acute infection in children.
4. Pelvic mass.
5. Retention of urine.
6. Pelvic pain.

> **Always scan both kidneys when examining the bladder.**

Preparation

1. **Preparation of the patient.** The bladder must be full. Give 4 or 5 glasses of fluid and examine after one hour (do not allow the patient to micturate). Alternatively, fill the bladder through a urethral catheter with sterile normal saline: stop when the patient feels uncomfortable. Avoid catheterization if possible because of the risk of infection.

1 litre

2. **Position of the patient.** The patient should lie supine but may need to be rotated obliquely.

   The patient should be relaxed, lying comfortably and breathing quietly.

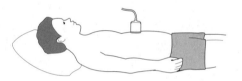

   Lubricate the lower abdomen with coupling agent. Hair anywhere on the abdomen will trap air bubbles so apply coupling agent generously.

3. **Choice of transducer.** Use a 3.5 MHz transducer for adults. Use a 5 MHz transducer for children or thin adults.

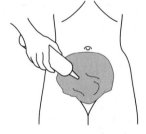
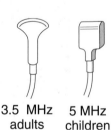

3.5 MHz adults   5 MHz children

Scanning technique

Start with transverse scans from the pubic symphysis upwards to the umbilicus. Follow with longitudinal scans, moving from one side of the lower abdomen to the other.

These scans will usually be sufficient, but it is not always easy to see the position of the lateral and anterior walls of the bladder and patients may have to be turned 30–45° to see an area more clearly. Any area that appears abnormal must be viewed in several projections. After scanning, the patient should empty the bladder and should then be rescanned.

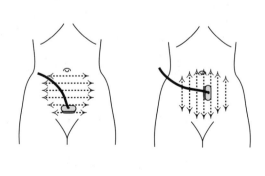

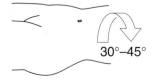

30°–45°

Normal bladder

The full urinary bladder appears as a large, echo-free area arising out of the pelvis. Start by assessing the smoothness of the interior wall of the bladder and its symmetry in transverse section. The thickness of the bladder wall will vary with the degree of distention but should always be approximately the same all around the bladder. Any local area of thickening is abnormal. Look also for trabeculation (see pp. 178–179). When distended, the normal bladder wall is less than 4 mm thick.

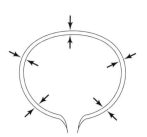

full bladder: wall less than 4 mm thick

After scanning, the patient should empty the bladder (Fig. 120c). Normally, there should be no residual urine: if there is, the quantity should be estimated. Measure the transverse diameter (T) of the bladder in centimetres, multiply it by the longitudinal diameter (L) in centimetres and then by the AP diameter in centimetres. Multiply the total by 0.52. This measures the residual urine in millilitres (cubic centimetres).

When the bladder has been thoroughly examined, scan the kidneys and the ureters (see Chapter 13).

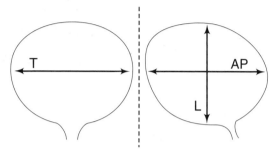

$T \times L \times AP \times 0.52 =$ volume (ml)

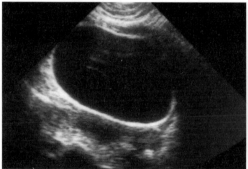
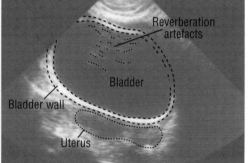

Fig. 120a. Longitudinal scan: normal full bladder.

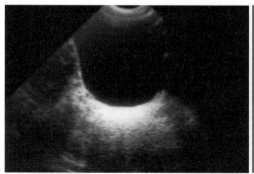
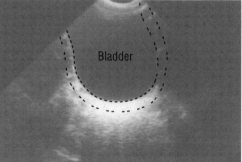

Fig. 120b. Transverse scan: normal full bladder.

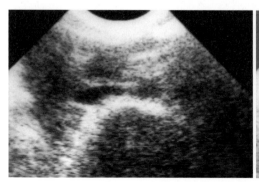
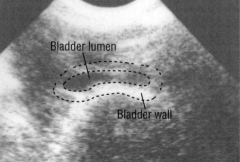

Fig. 120c. Transverse scan: normal empty bladder.

Abnormal bladder

It is important to scan for:

1. Variation of the bladder wall thickness and trabeculation.

2. Asymmetry of the bladder.

3. Cystic masses within the bladder (ureterocele or diverticulum).

4. Solid masses within the bladder or at the base of the bladder.

For differential diagnosis, see pp. 182–183.

Generalized thickening of the bladder wall

1. In men, bladder wall thickening is usually the result of prostatic obstruction (Fig. 121a). If suspected, check the prostate (Fig. 124c, p. 183): exclude hydronephrosis by scanning the ureter and the kidneys. Search for associated diverticula: these project outwards but are only visible if over 1 cm in diameter. Diverticula are usually echo-free with good sound transmission (Fig. 121b). Sometimes the opening of a diverticulum can be demonstrated: diverticula may collapse or increase in size after micturition.

2. Severe, chronic infection/cystitis. The inner wall of the bladder may be thickened and irregular (Fig. 121c). Check the rest of the renal tract for dilatation.

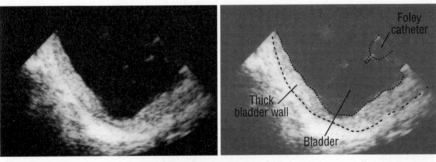

Fig. 121a. Hypertrophy of the wall of the bladder.

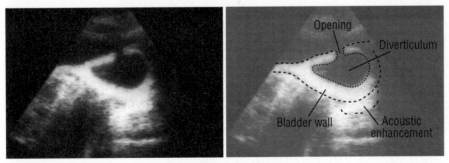

Fig. 121b. Longitudinal scan: diverticulum of the bladder.

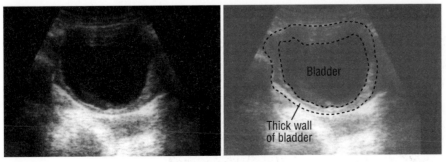

Fig. 121c. Chronic bladder infection (chronic cystitis).

3. Schistosomiasis. The bladder walls may be thickened, with increased echogenicity and scattered dense (bright) areas due to calcification (Fig. 122a, b). The calcification varies and may be throughout or patchy, and differing in thickness. The calcification is in the intramural ova and does not prevent normal contraction of the bladder.

   Poor bladder emptying indicates superimposed active infection, or prolonged or recurrent infection. The extent of the calcification does not indicate the activity of the schistosomal infection, and calcification may decrease in the later stages. However, the bladder wall usually remains thickened and does not easily distend. There may also be hydronephrosis (Fig. 122c).

4. Very thick trabeculated bladder walls in children may result from outlet obstruction caused by urethral valves or urogenital diaphragm.

5. A thickened bladder wall may occur in a neurogenic bladder and will usually be associated with uretero-hydronephrosis.

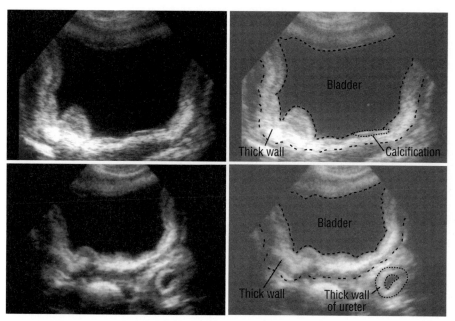

Fig. 122a. Two transverse scans showing thickening and irregularity of the bladder wall of a 12-year-old child with schistosomiasis. The left ureter is also thickened (lower).

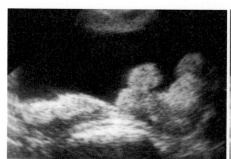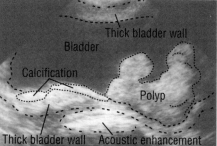

Fig. 122b. Transverse scan: marked polypoid mucosal thickening and patchy calcification in the bladder of an 8-year-old child with schistosomiasis.

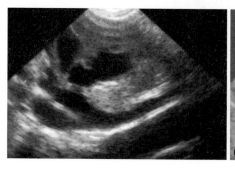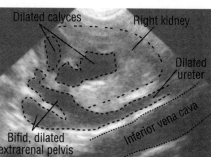

Fig. 122c. Longitudinal scan: hydronephrosis and hydroureter caused by schistosomiasis. There is also sludge in the renal pelvis as a result of associated urinary tract infection.

Localized thickening of the bladder wall

Whenever localized bladder wall thickening is suspected, multidirectional scans are needed, particularly to exclude a polyp. Moving the patient or increasing the volume of fluid in the bladder will help to identify bladder folds. (Folds will disappear as the bladder distends.) If there is any doubt, repeat after 1 or 2 hours: do not let the patient micturate before the examination is repeated (Fig. 123a, b).

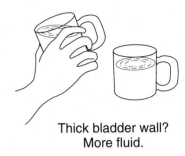

Thick bladder wall?
More fluid.

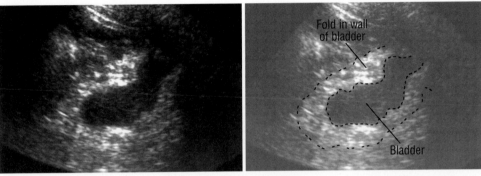

Fig. 123a. Longitudinal scan: apparent thickening with folds in the wall of a partially filled bladder.

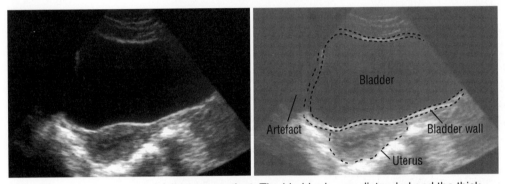

Fig. 123b. Transverse scan of the same patient. The bladder is now distended and the thick folds have disappeared.

Localized thickening may be due to:

1. Bladder fold due to incomplete filling (Fig. 123 a, b).

2. Tumour: sessile or polypoid, single or multiple (Fig. 123c, d, e).

3. Localized infection due to tuberculosis or to schistosomal plaques (granulomas) (Fig. 122a, c, p. 179).

4. Acute reaction to schistosomal infection in children.

5. Haematoma following trauma (Fig. 123f).

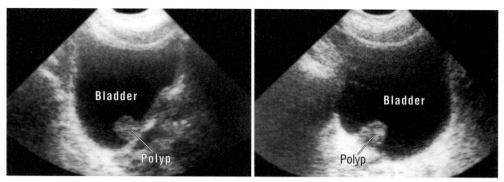

Fig. 123c. A sessile polyp in the bladder: longitudinal (left) and transverse (right) scans.

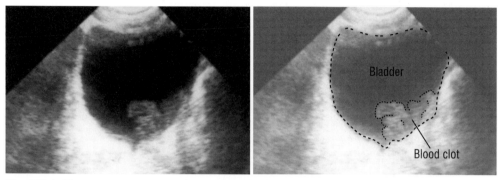

Fig. 123d. Transverse scan: pseudotumour in the bladder, caused by blood clots.

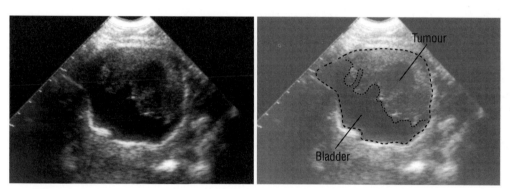

Fig. 123e. Transverse scan: a large malignant tumour arising from the bladder wall.

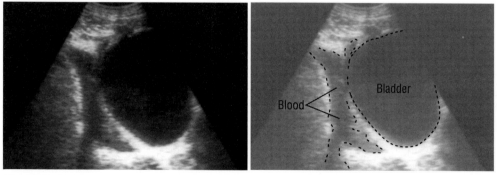

Fig. 123f. Transverse scan: following injury, there is blood lateral to the bladder, distorting and apparently thickening the bladder wall.

Differential diagnosis of localized bladder wall thickening

1. Most bladder neoplasms are multiple but located in one area. Some only thicken the bladder wall, but most are also polypoid. It is essential to recognize when the tumour has spread through the bladder wall. Calcification in the tumour or wall due to associated schistosomiasis may cause bright echoes (Fig. 122 and 123, pp. 179 and 181).

2. Bladder polyps are often mobile on a stalk, but some, especially those due to infection, may be sessile and not easily differentiated from a malignant tumour (Fig. 123c, p. 181).

3. Granulomas (e.g. tuberculous) cause multifocal but localized thickening. The bladder is often small and becomes painful when distended, resulting in frequent micturition: in malignancy, bladder distention is painless. Schistosomiasis may cause multiple flat plaques and polyps (Fig. 122, p. 179). Any chronic infection will eventually decrease bladder capacity (see p. 186).

4. Trauma. If there is localized thickening following trauma, scan the pelvis to exclude fluid (blood or urine) outside the bladder (Fig. 123f, p. 181). Repeat the scan after 10–14 days. If the thickening is due to a haematoma, the swelling should have decreased.

5. Schistosomiasis. Children who are reinfected can have an acute "urticarial" reaction in the bladder wall causing marked local thickening of the bladder mucosa. This subsides with treatment or spontaneously over a few weeks (Fig. 122a, p. 179).

> **Blood clot and tumour look alike, and both may be associated with haematuria.**

Density within the bladder

1. **Attached to the wall**

   - Polyp. A polyp on a long stalk may appear freely mobile. Change the patient's position and rescan.

   - Adherent calculus. Calculi can be single or multiple, small or large: they usually have acoustic shadowing. Some may become adherent to the bladder mucosa, especially when there is infection: scan with the patient in different positions to assess movement (Fig. 124a) (see also p. 184).

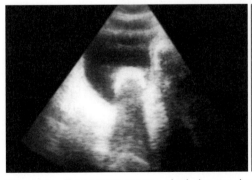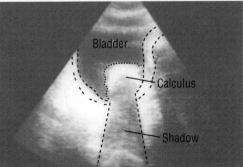

Fig. 124a. Transverse scan: a single large calculus adherent to the bladder wall.

- Ureterocele. A ureterocele presents as a cystic mass within the bladder, near a ureteric orifice (Fig. 124b). It will change in size if scanned at different times. In children, the ureterocele may be so large that the opposite ureter is also obstructed. Ureteroceles are sometimes bilateral but are seldom symmetrical. If suspected, scan the kidneys and the ureters for asymmetrical hydronephrosis and hydroureter, and for duplication of the ureters (p. 159).

- Enlarged prostate. An echogenic, non-mobile mass located centrally at the base of the bladder in a male patient is most likely an enlarged prostate (Fig. 124c). In women, an enlarged uterus can also distort the bladder (Fig. 124d).

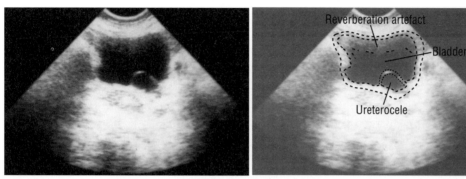

Fig. 124b. Transverse scan: a prominent ureterocele.

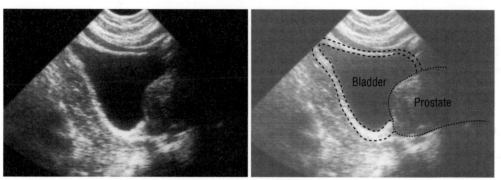

Fig. 124c. Longitudinal scan: a markedly enlarged prostate.

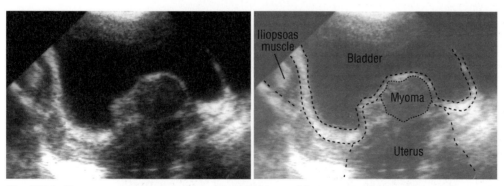

Fig. 124d. Transverse scan: distortion of the bladder wall by pressure from a large uterine myoma.

2. **Mobile density within the bladder**

- Calculus. Unless they are very large, most calculi move within the bladder (Fig. 125a). However, calculi may be trapped in a diverticulum or be so large that they seem to fill the bladder: the capacity of the bladder to hold urine will be reduced when there is a large stone. When there is doubt about a bladder calculus, change the position of the patient and rescan. Most small and medium-size calculi will change position, but a large calculus may not be able to move (Fig. 124a, p. 182).

- Foreign body. Catheters must be recognized (Fig. 125b). Very rarely a foreign body is introduced into the bladder. If this is suspected, a careful history is necessary: X-rays may be helpful.

- Blood clot. A thrombus can resemble a calculus or a foreign body: not all blood clots are freely mobile (Fig. 125c).

- Air. Introduced into the bladder either through a catheter or by infection or through a fistula, air appears as an echogenic, mobile, non-dependent (floating) area.

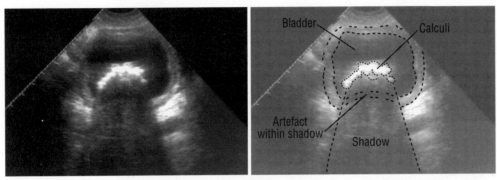

Fig. 125a. Transverse scan: multiple calculi in the bladder.

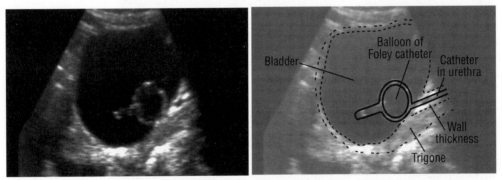

Fig. 125b. Longitudinal scan: the balloon of a Foley catheter next to the bladder wall.

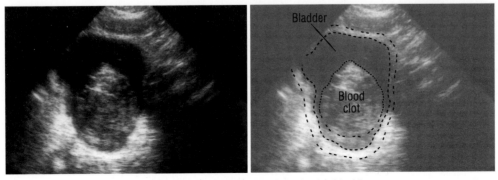

Fig. 125c. Transverse scan: a large, laminated blood clot in the bladder.

Large (overdistended) bladder

When distended, the bladder walls will be smooth and evenly stretched, with or without diverticula Use measurements to confirm suspected overdistension (Fig. 126a, b).

Always look at the ureters and check the kidneys for hydronephrosis. Ask the patient to empty the bladder and rescan to see if it is completely empty (Fig. 126c).

Common causes of bladder distention are:

1. Enlargement of the prostate.
2. Urethral stricture in the male.
3. Urethral calculus in the male.
4. Bruising of the urethra in the female ("honeymoon urethritis").
5. A neurogenic bladder from damage to the spinal cord.
6. Urethral valves or diaphragm in newborn infants.
7. Cystocele in some patients.

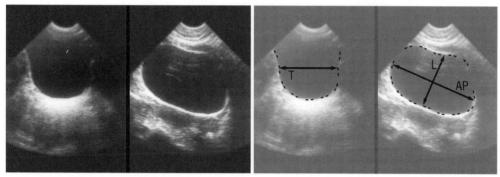

Fig. 126a. Normal full bladder and measurements: transverse scan (left) and longitudinal scan (right). Volume (ml) = T × L × AP × 0.52

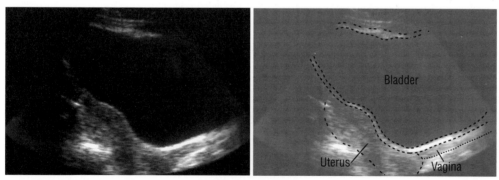

Fig. 126b. Longitudinal scan: an overdistended bladder.

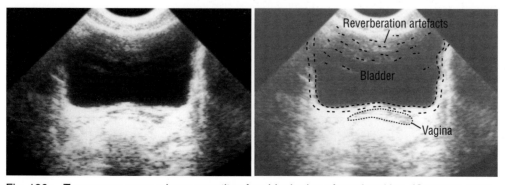

Fig. 126c. Transverse scan: a large quantity of residual urine after micturition. (Compare empty bladder, Fig. 120c, p. 177).

Small bladder

A bladder may be small because of cystitis, which prevents the patient from holding urine and causes a clinical history of frequent and painful micturition. The bladder may also be small because the walls have been damaged or fibrosed, reducing the bladder capacity (Fig. 127). Micturition will then be frequent but not painful.

If there is any doubt, give the patient more fluid and ask him or her not to micturate; rescan in 1–2 hours.

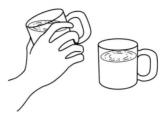

Small bladder?
More fluid

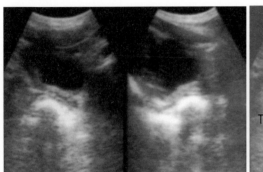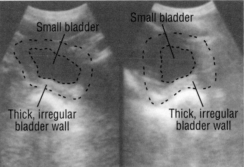

Fig. 127. Longitudinal scans in different planes: the bladder is small and irregular as a result of fibrosis. It did not distend any further, even after the patient had drunk more fluid.

A small bladder may be due to:

1. Late schistosomiasis. There may be bright echoes due to calcification (see p. 179).

2. Recurrent cystitis, particularly due to tuberculosis. Bladder wall thickening is likely (Fig. 121c, p. 178).

3. The rare infiltrating neoplasm. When there is a tumour, the bladder wall is nearly always asymmetrical (see p. 182).

4. Radiotherapy or surgery for malignancy. Check the clinical history.

> **Always ask the patient to drink more fluid and rescan in 1–2 hours before diagnosing a small bladder.**

CHAPTER 15

Scrotum and testis

Indications

1. Swelling of the scrotum.
2. Trauma.
3. Infection.
4. Pain.
5. Apparently absent testicle (swelling in the groin in young males).
6. Haematospermia.
7. Infertility.

Preparation

1. **Preparation of the patient**. No preparation is required.
2. **Position of the patient**. The patient should be supine. Lift the penis upwards towards the abdomen and cover with a towel.

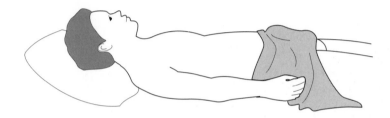

   Apply coupling agent liberally to cover the scrotum.
3. **Choice of transducer**. If available, a 7.5 MHz sector transducer is preferable, especially for children. Otherwise, use a 5 MHz transducer.

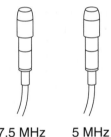

7.5 MHz   5 MHz

Scanning technique

Scan both testes from different angles. Compare the testes at each projection.

The normal testis

The normal testis is oval, homogeneous and hyperechogenic (Fig. 128a, b).

1. The average length in the adult is 5.0 cm.

2. The average width is 3.0 cm.

3. The average transverse diameter is 2.0 cm.

4. The vertical diameter is 2.5 cm.

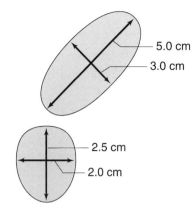

The epididymis lies on the inferior aspect of the testis and is more echogenic than the testis. It is subdivided into a head, body and tail, the head being the part most reliably demonstrated by ultrasound (Fig. 128c).

The two testes are separated in the scrotum by a hyperechogenic septum. There are often small collections of fluid within the scrotum.

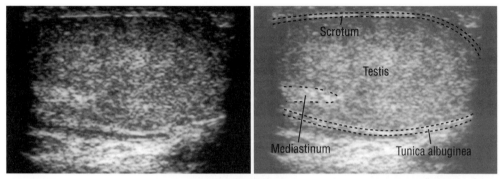

Fig. 128a. Longitudinal scan: normal testis. The fibrous testicular mediastinum can be identified.

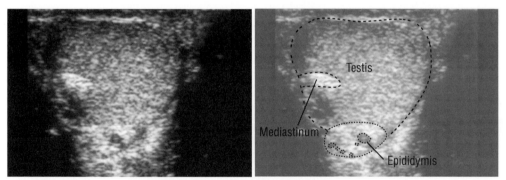

Fig. 128b. Transverse scan: normal testis.

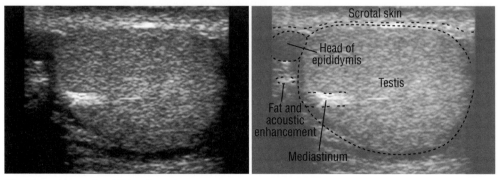

Fig.128c. Normal epididymis and scrotum.

Abnormal scrotum

Unilateral swelling

Swelling on one side of the scrotum may be due to:

1. **Hydrocele**. Fluid in the scrotum will surround the testis with an echo-free region, varying in size and position (Fig. 129). If the fluid is due to inflammation or trauma, there may be internal debris causing internal echoes on ultrasound. The testis must be carefully examined to exclude underlying malignancy (Fig. 130).

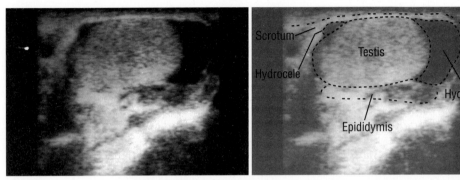

Fig. 129a. Longitudinal scan: a small hydrocele.

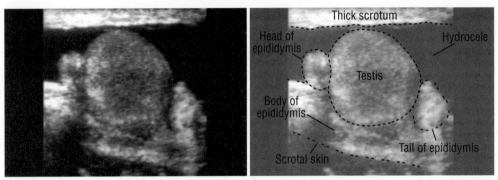

Fig.129b. Longitudinal scan: a moderate hydrocele.

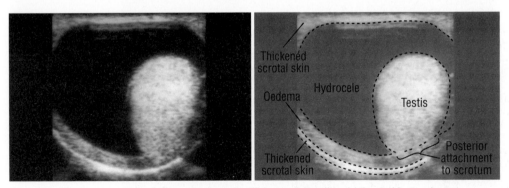

Fig.129c. Transverse scan: a large hydrocele. The scrotal wall is thickened by oedema.

2. **Trauma and torsion of the testis** (see p. 193).
3. **Hernia** (see p. 194).
4. **Varicocele** (see p. 194).

5. **Testicular mass**, e.g. tumour or infection. The majority of testicular tumours are malignant. The tumours may be hypoechogenic or hyperechogenic, and the testis may be normal in size or enlarged. The two testes must be compared, because a tumour may replace all the normal tissue, and can then only be recognized by the difference in echogenicity. Even when the two testes are of equal density, gentle compression may show a small tumour not demonstrated by routine scanning (Fig. 130a, b). It can be difficult to distinguish between tumour and infection (Fig 130c).

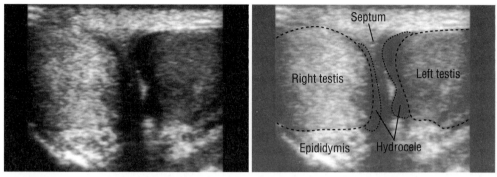

Fig.130a. Transverse scans: the right testis is normal; the left testis is hypoechogenic. This could be because of infection or oedema associated with a small tumour. There is a bilateral hydrocele, the left larger than the right.

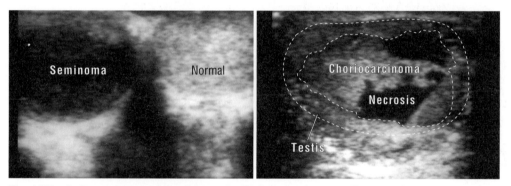

Fig. 130b. Left: seminoma of the right testis. Right: mixed germ cell tumour (choriocarcinoma) of the left testis with areas of necrosis.

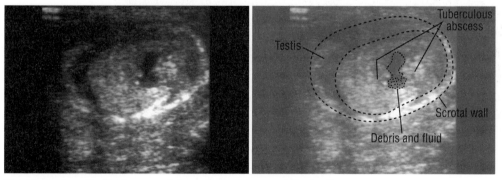

Fig. 130c. Longitudinal scan: a tuberculous abscess of the testis.

Small or absent testis

Failure to demonstrate a testis in the scrotum with ultrasound indicates that the testis is absent. If clinical examination of the inguinal canal reveals a mass, ultrasound can demonstrate the location and size of the mass, but may not be able to differentiate testicular tissue from an enlarged lymph node. If there is no palpable mass in the inguinal region on clinical examination, there is no indication to proceed with ultrasound.

The epididymis

The epididymis may become infected or develop cysts.

1. **Epididymitis**. Ultrasound will demonstrate an enlarged and hypoechogenic epididymis on the affected side. If there is associated orchitis, the testis will also be comparatively hypoechogenic (Fig. 131a, b). Chronic epididymitis may have both hypo- and hyperechogenic areas (Fig. 131c.)

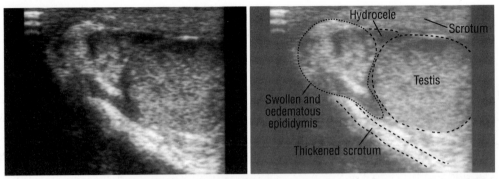

Fig. 131a. Transverse scan: acute epididymitis.

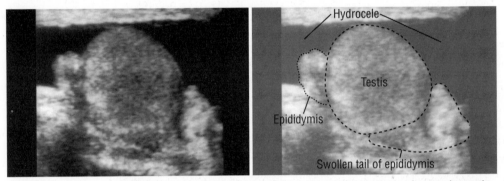

Fig. 131b. Moderate epididymo-orchitis; both the epididymis and the testis are hypoechogenic and swollen. There is a hydrocele.

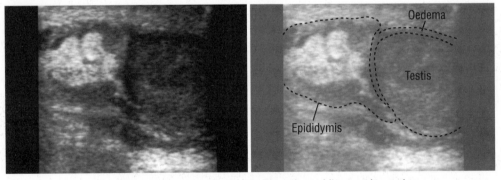

Fig. 131c. Chronic epididymitis. There are hypoechogenic and hyperechogenic areas.

2. **Cyst in the epididymis**. Cysts may be single or multiple, and are confined to the epididymis. The testis will not be affected. Epididymal cysts must be differentiated from the more tubular varicocele (see p. 194).

Trauma

Following injury, the testis may be enlarged or remain normal in size. When there is excess fluid in the scrotum, the testis should be scanned at many diferent angles to exclude rupture. The injured testis may show complex echogenicity, especially when there is an internal haematoma (or subsequent abscess). Blood will appear as fluid within the scrotum, often with complex echogenicity due to blood clots (Fig. 132a, b).

Torsion of the testis

It may be difficult to confirm torsion of the testis with ultrasound, but if the rotation has disrupted the normal blood supply, ultrasound will demonstrate decreased echogenicity, compared with the normal testis, in the acute stage (Fig.132c). There may be associated scrotal fluid (hydrocele) (see also p. 190).

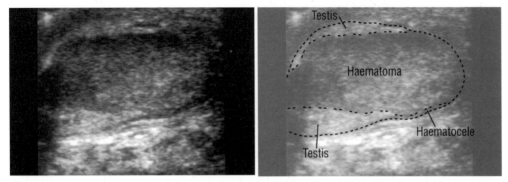

Fig. 132a. Longitudinal scan: a haematoma of the testis without disruption (fracture) but with a small haematocele.

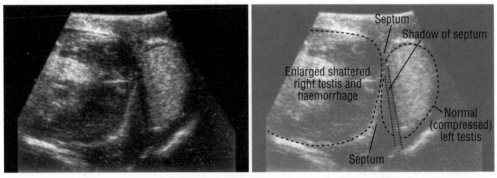

Fig. 132b. Transverse scan. Shattered and swollen right testis, with compression of the left testis. There is a small haematocele.

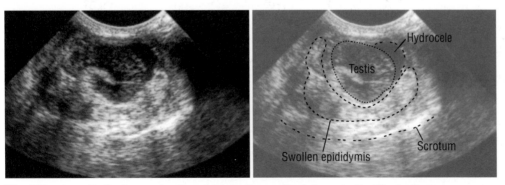

Fig. 132c. Longitudinal scan: torsion of the testis, confirmed surgically. The testis has decreased echogenicity.

Hernia

Omenta, mesentery or intestinal loops that have prolapsed through an inguinal hernia into the scrotum are usually associated with a small hydrocele. The loops of bowel will appear on ultrasound as a complex mass within the echo-free fluid. If there is a significant solid content within the bowel, there will be hyperechogenic areas also (Fig. 133).

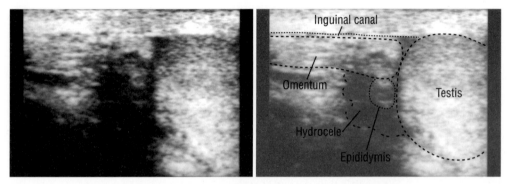

Fig. 133. Longitudinal scan: a small inguinal hernia in a young, healthy male.

Varicocele

When the veins draining the testis and epididymis are dilated, ultrasound will demonstrate multiple tortuous, tubular, hypoechogenic structures around the periphery of the testis, which is often smaller than the normal testis (Fig. 134a). Varicocele is more common on the left side: there may be associated infertility. The underlying testis must be scanned to exclude a tumour and varicocele must be differentiated from spermatocele (Fig. 134b). A Valsalva manoeuvre will often cause the veins to dilate.

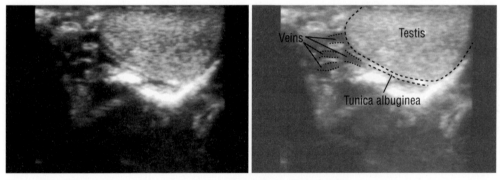

Fig. 134a. Transverse scan: a varicocele with multiple dilated veins.

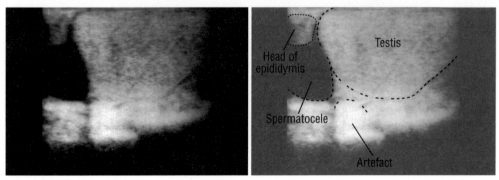

Fig. 134b. Transverse scan: a spermatocele.

CHAPTER 16

Gynaecology (non-pregnant female pelvis)

Indications

1. Pelvic pain, including dysmenorrhoea (painful menstruation).
2. Pelvic mass.
3. Abnormal vaginal bleeding.
4. Abnormal vaginal discharge.
5. Amenorrhoea (missed or absent menstrual cycle).
6. To confirm the presence and check the position of an intrauterine contraceptive device.
7. Infertility: hysterosalpingography may also be needed.
8. Genital tract developmental abnormality: hysterosalpingography may also be needed.
9. Urinary or bladder symptoms (see also Chapter 14).
10. Diffuse abdominal pain.
11. Follicular monitoring in investigation of infertility.

> **Ultrasound does not demonstrate the anatomy of vesico-vaginal fistula. It may help to exclude complications.**

Preparation

1. **Preparation of the patient**. The bladder must be full. Give 4 or 5 glasses of fluid and examine after one hour (do not allow the patient to micturate). Alternatively, fill the bladder through a urethral catheter with sterile normal saline: stop when the patient feels uncomfortable. Avoid catheterization if possible because of the risk of infection.

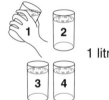

1 litre total

2. **Position of the patient**. The patient is usually scanned while lying comfortably on her back (supine). It may be necessary to rotate the patient after the preliminary scans. Erect scanning is occasionally needed.

   Apply coupling agent liberally to the lower abdomen: it is not usually necessary to cover the pubic hair, but, if required, apply freely.

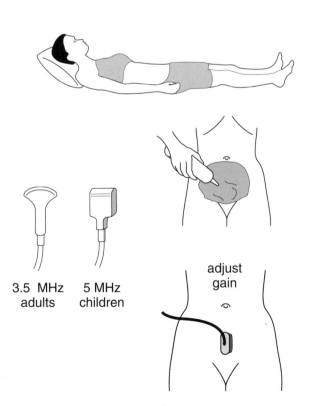

3. **Choice of transducer**. Use a 3.5 MHz transducer for adults. Use a 5 MHz transducer for children or thin adults.

   3.5 MHz adults   5 MHz children

4. **Setting the correct gain**. Position the transducer longitudinally over the full bladder and adjust the gain to produce the best image.

   adjust gain

Scanning technique

Start with longitudinal scans, first in the midline between the umbilicus and the pubic symphysis. Then, repeat more laterally, first on the left side and then on the right. Angle the transducer from side to side and longitudinally to identify the uterus.

Next, scan transversely. Start just above the pubic symphysis and move upwards to the umbilicus. Transverse scans are important over the lower pelvis but are less effective above the level of the uterus.

If necessary, turn the patient obliquely (30–40°) to identify the ovaries. Scan each ovary obliquely, from the contralateral side of the abdomen (see also pp. 204–209).

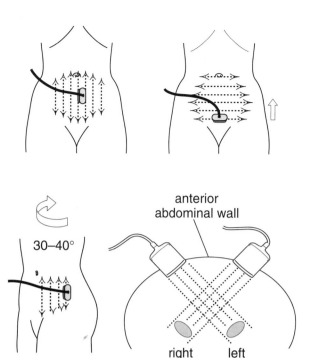

to identify ovaries

anterior abdominal wall

right ovary left ovary

Endovaginal ultrasound

A different and specific transducer with a long handle is needed to perform ultrasound from the vagina: specialized training is necessary. Put sufficient coupling agent inside a condom or other disposable plastic cover to provide good contact: the cover also prevents infection. *Do **not** use any other transducer or any uncovered transducer.*

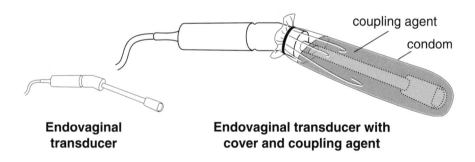

coupling agent

condom

Endovaginal transducer

Endovaginal transducer with cover and coupling agent

With this technique, the bladder must be *empty*.

The field of view by endovaginal sonography is much smaller and considerable experience is needed both to obtain satisfactory images and to interpret them. The technique is very useful for imaging an early pregnancy and some uterine, fallopian tube or ovarian masses (including ectopic pregnancy).

Endovaginal sonography can be misleading if the operator is not well trained.

Normal anatomy

Locate the vagina and the uterus on a longitudinal scan. The vagina is close to the postero–inferior wall of the urinary bladder and the walls of the vagina will appear as hypoechogenic structures surrounding the more echogenic vaginal mucosa (Fig. 135a). Follow the vagina superiorly and the tissues will expand into the pear-shaped uterus, superior to the vagina but with different echogenicity (varying with the phase of the menstrual cycle) (see p. 212). Adjustment of the gain may be necessary during these initial scans to obtain the best image.

The uterus has two different zones of echogenicity. The muscles in the uterine wall are hypoechogenic, but the pattern of the endometrium varies (Fig. 135b). In the first half of the menstrual cycle (post-menstruation) the endometrium is thin and hypoechogenic. In the second half, the premenstrual phase, the endometrium is hyperechogenic (see also Fig. 148, p. 212).

The uterus may not be exactly in the long axis of the pelvis and may be seen tangentially. The long axis of the uterus is measured from fundus to cervix.

The normal postpubertal nulliparous uterus measures 4.5–9.0 cm in length, 1.5–3 cm antero–posteriorly, and 4.5–5.5 cm in the transverse diameter. Uterine dimensions increase by 1.0–1.2 cm with parity, and the body of the uterus becomes more rounded (Fig. 140, p. 202). The antero–posterior diameter of the uterine cervix should not exceed the antero–posterior diameter of the uterine body (for measurements in children, see p. 199).

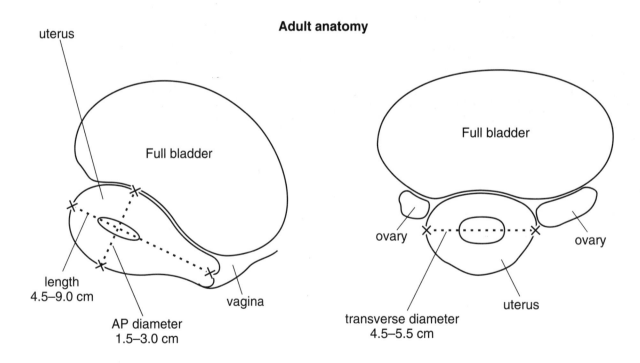

Adult anatomy

uterus

Full bladder

length
4.5–9.0 cm

vagina

AP diameter
1.5–3.0 cm

Full bladder

ovary

ovary

uterus

transverse diameter
4.5–5.5 cm

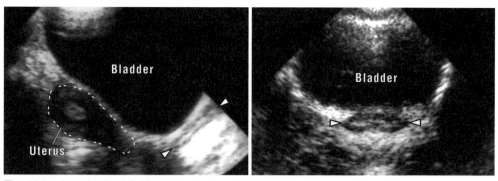

Fig. 135a. Longitudinal (left) and transverse (right) scans of a normal vagina (arrows).

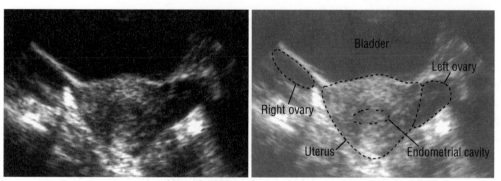

Fig. 135b. Longitudinal scan of a normal uterus.

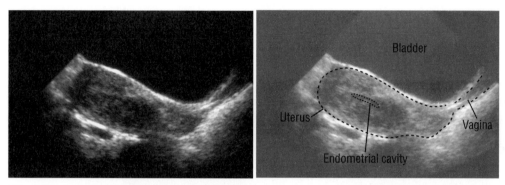

Fig. 135c. Transverse scan of a normal uterus.

The pre-pubertal uterus

As the child grows, the ratio of the uterine cervix to the uterine body changes. In childhood the body of the uterus is smaller than the cervix, but with increasing age, the uterine body grows larger and the endometrium is not demonstrated.

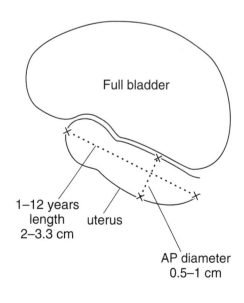

Vagina, rectum and bladder

Transverse scans should start with steep angulation posteriorly and downwards. Identify the vagina, the rectum and the lower part of the urinary bladder. Examine the shape of the bladder at this level. Keeping the transducer in the midline, slowly sweep the scan plane from the bottom to the top of the pelvic cavity (Fig. 135, p. 199).

Identify the junction of the vagina with the cervix of the uterus, then the ligament on either side of the cervix, the narrow "neck" (isthmus) and the body of the uterus. Look for both ovaries (see pp. 204–208).

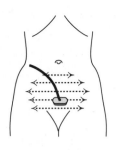

The normal echo pattern of the vagina may be altered by a tampon (Fig. 136a, b) or foreign objects, such as a pessary (Fig. 136c).

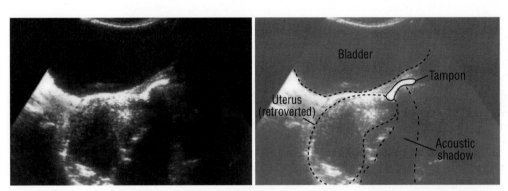

Fig. 136a. Longitudinal scan: a tampon in the vagina. (The uterus is retroverted; see p. 203).

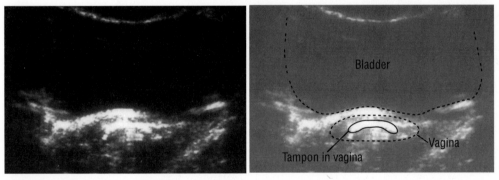

Fig. 136b. Transverse scan of the same patient.

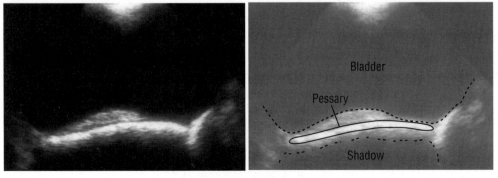

Fig. 136c. Transverse scan: a pessary in the posterior vaginal fornix with an acoustic shadow below it.

Intrauterine contraceptive device

An intrauterine contraceptive device (IUD) will appear as a linear or interrupted hyperechogenic line within the endometrial cavity or cervical canal and may produce distal acoustic shadowing (Fig. 137) (see also p. 229).

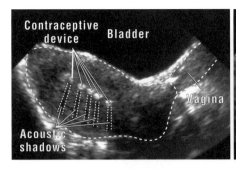
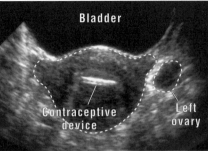

Fig. 137a. Longitudinal (left) and transverse (right) scans: an intrauterine contraceptive device causing acoustic shadows.

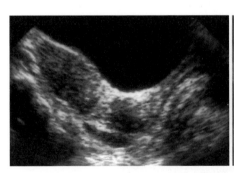
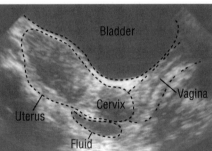

Fig. 137b. Longitudinal scan: an IUD in the cervical canal, extending into the vagina.

Fluid in the posterior cul-de-sac

It is not unusual to find a small amount of fluid in the posterior cul-de-sac following ovulation or menstruation (Fig. 138). An echo-free cross-sectional diameter of less than 1 cm is normal.

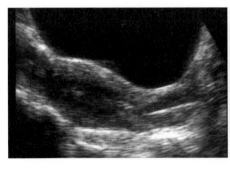
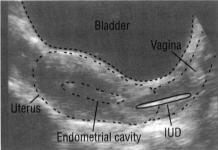

Fig. 138a. Longitudinal section showing a small amount of fluid in the cul-de-sac; this is normal after ovulation or menstruation.

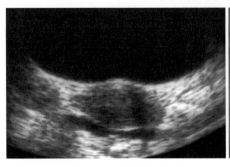
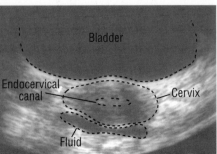

Fig. 138b. Transverse scan of the same patient.

Uterine cervix

Scan the uterine cervix in different projections and note any abnormal variation in size or shape (Fig. 139a). After pregnancy the cervix may be asymmetrical (Fig. 139b).

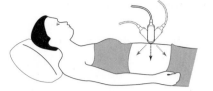

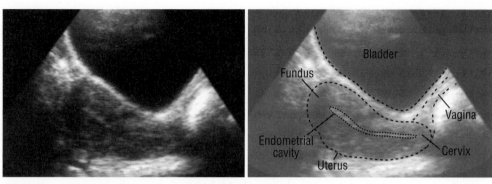

Fig. 139a. Longitudinal scan: the normal uterine cervix.

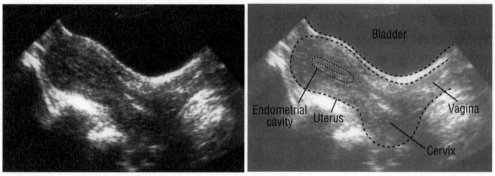

Fig. 139b. Longitudinal scan: a multiparous cervix.

Following each pregnancy, the uterus increases in size and the body of the uterus becomes more rounded. Thus, the uterus of a multiparous patient (Fig. 140) will look quite different from that of a nulliparous patient. Record the uterine dimensions. (See also pp. 198, 199.)

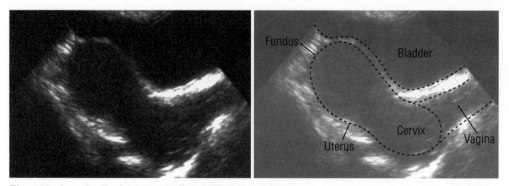

Fig. 140. Longitudinal scan: a bulky multiparous uterus.

The postmenopausal pelvis

1. Uterus. After the menopause the uterus is much smaller and will appear homogeneous: the endometrial cavity will not be visible.

2. Ovaries after the menopause. The ovaries are small and often very difficult or impossible to recognize with ultrasound. If seen, they are hyperechogenic, without any follicles and similar to the surrounding tissues.

Position of the uterus

The uterus may rotate so that the fundus of the uterus may be behind the cervix (retroversion). It may also rotate forward (anteversion).

If the body of the uterus bends forward at the cervix, it is anteflexed (Fig. 141a). When the uterus bends backwards at the cervix, it is retroflexed (Fig. 141b).

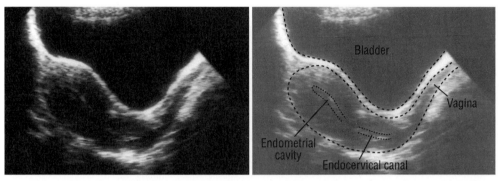

Fig. 141a. Longitudinal scan: an anteflexed uterus, which bends forward at the cervix and lifts the posterior bladder wall.

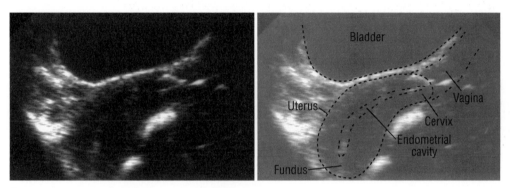

Fig. 141b. Longitudinal scan: a retroflexed uterus.

If the uterus is not identified, check the patient's surgical history to exclude a hysterectomy. When there has been pelvic surgery, look carefully for the remnants of the cervix, suggesting a partial hysterectomy (Fig. 141c) (see also p. 207 for useful scanning techniques).

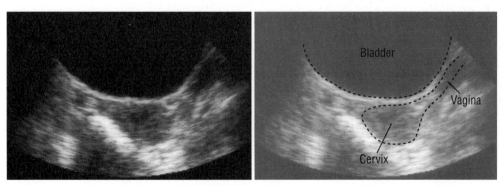

Fig. 141c. Longitudinal scan: only the uterine cervix is seen; the body of the uterus has been surgically removed (partial hysterectomy).

When normal pelvic anatomy is not clearly recognized, give the patient more fluid to fill the bladder (see pp. 206–207).

Ovaries

Scan the tissues on the left close to the uterus. Angle the transducer as required to locate the left ovary, which will appear as an ovoid (egg-shaped) structure, less homogeneous than the uterus but with the same or slightly less echogenicity: there will often be distal acoustic shadowing (Fig. 142a).

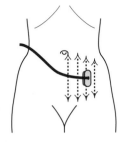

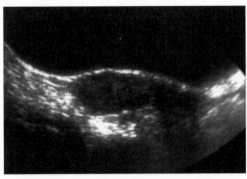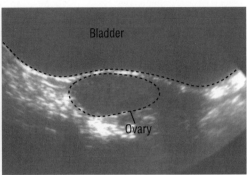

Fig. 142a. Longitudinal scan: normal left ovary.

The ovaries can vary in position but always lie behind the bladder and the uterus. They are most commonly found in the adnexal space laterally (Fig. 142b).

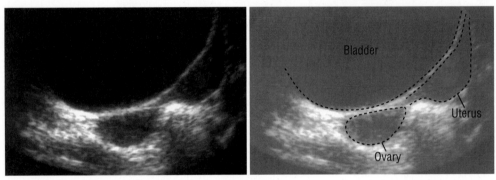

Fig. 142b. Angled transverse scan: normal right ovary.

An ovary may be located in the cul-de-sac or cephalad to the fundus of the uterus (Fig. 142c). In postmenopausal women, the ovaries are small and may be difficult to identify.

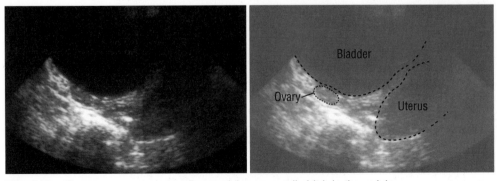

Fig. 142c. Transverse scan: a small ovary lying unusually high in the pelvis.

If it is difficult to differentiate between the uterus and the ovaries, move the uterus manually per vagina and continue to scan, using different projections and positions to clarify the anatomy. The same technique can be used when there is a lower pelvic mass (see also p. 207).

When the ovaries cannot be identified, the following techniques may be helpful:

1. Turn the patient obliquely and scan the opposite ovary through the full bladder (Fig. 142d).

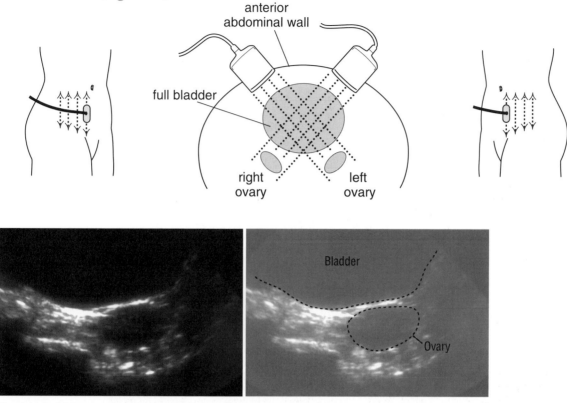

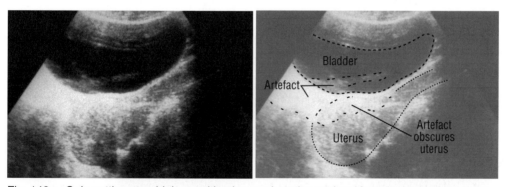

Fig. 142d. Oblique scan: the ovary is seen through the bladder.

2. Reduce the gain settings. If the gain is set too high, the ovary may blend into the surrounding parametrium and be difficult to identify (Fig. 142e, f).

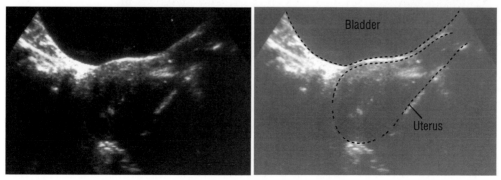

Fig. 142e. Gain settings too high, resulting in reverberation and artefacts in the bladder and poor definition of the uterus.

Fig. 142f. Gain setting too low, so that the posterior portion of the uterus is not clearly seen.

If the ovaries are still difficult to identify, there may be too much or too little urine in the bladder. If the bladder does not extend to the level of the uterine fundus, it is probably not full enough and the patient should drink more water (Fig. 143). Rescan 30 minutes later: if the bladder is then full enough, try to identify the ovaries.

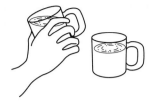

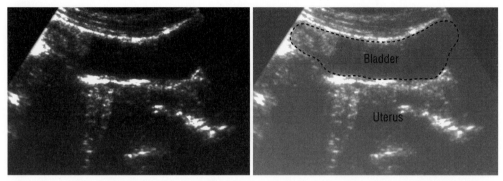

Fig. 143a. Inadequate filling of the bladder, which does not cover the uterus, making it difficult to see.

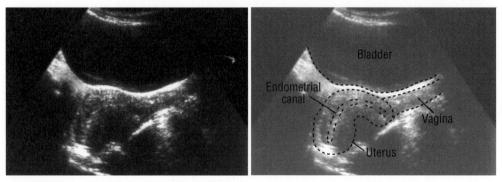

Fig. 143b. The bladder of the same patient is now properly filled and extends past the fundus of the retroverted uterus.

If the bladder is overfilled, it will push the ovaries against the uterus or laterally onto the psoas muscle. Ask the patient to partially empty the bladder (give her a specific measure, such as a small jug or bowl to fill). Then repeat the scan.

Even when the bladder is correctly filled, the ovaries may be difficult to image because of overlying bowel gas. This is particularly important if the ovary lies higher in the pelvis than usual (Fig. 143c).

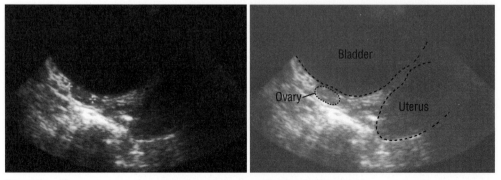

Fig. 143c. Transverse scan: an ovary lying unusually high in the pelvis.

If necessary, scan the patient in the erect and oblique-erect positions. This may displace the gas-filled loops of bowel and allow the ovaries to be seen more clearly.

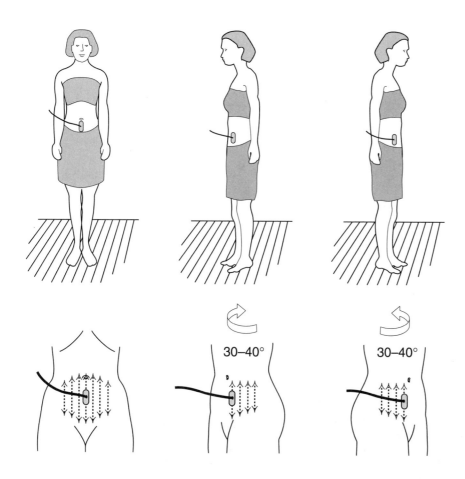

If the normal pelvic anatomy cannot be demonstrated, gently insert 20 ml of water at body temperature into the vagina while scanning above the pubic symphysis. The fluid will surround the cervix and simplify recognition. This procedure is particularly helpful in differentiating between partial and total hysterectomy when not possible by clinical examination.

If it is difficult to locate a retrouterine mass, insert 200 ml of warm water into the rectum while continuing to image the area. Microbubbles in the water will appear as strongly reflective echoes which will delineate the anterior wall of the rectum, and allow recognition of intraluminal masses, such as faeces, which are a common source of error.

Normal ovaries

When the ovaries have been found, check for displacement of any surrounding structure. Check the normal echo pattern and look for any distal acoustic enhancement. If there are anechoic spaces within or on the surface of the ovary, these are probably ovarian follicles (see p. 209). Reduce the gain when scanning the ovary because normal ovarian tissue transmits the echoes and enhances the deep tissues. Measure the size of each ovary (Fig. 144).

Examine the tissue around the ovary for cystic, solid or fluid-filled masses. Look particularly for fluid in the cul-de-sac. Examine both ovaries.

An ovary should not normally be found in front of the uterus. If it is in an abnormal position, rotate the patient to see if it is fixed by adhesions and note whether it is significantly enlarged.

As already noted, the gain setting must be varied while scanning the pelvis to obtain the best images (Fig. 142e, f, p. 205). The relationship of the pelvic organs may be more easily seen by slow, continuous scans, taking about 10 seconds.

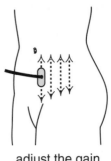

adjust the gain

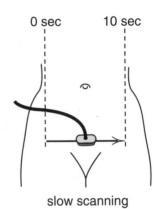

slow scanning

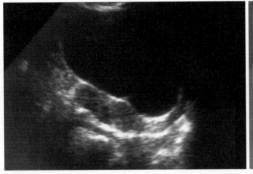 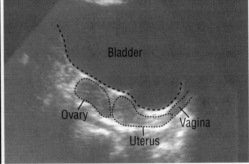

Fig. 144a. Longitudinal scan: a normal right ovary.

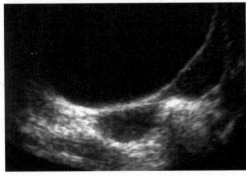 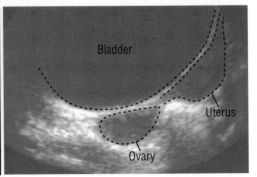

Fig. 144b. Transverse scan: a normal right ovary.

Ovarian follicles

Follicles normally show as cyst-like anechogenic spaces within or around the surface of the ovary and are best seen when the gain is low. Depending upon the phase of the menstrual cycle, the cyst may be up to 2.5 cm in diameter. Simple cysts measuring less than 5 cm may be physiological and will change, become smaller or disappear (Fig. 145).

If there is concern that a cyst is neoplastic, the patient should be scanned both early and late in the menstrual cycle. Follicular cysts should regress and nonfunctional cysts should not change in size. Scan after another month if still in doubt (see also p. 216).

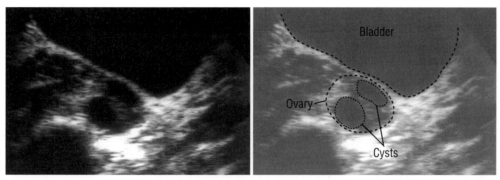

Fig. 145a. Longitudinal scan: two follicular cysts within the ovary.

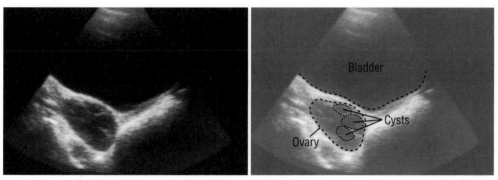

Fig. 145b. Longitudinal scan: an ovary with several surface follicular cysts.

A physiological cyst in the ovary may be up to 5 cm in diameter. Cysts of this size should be re-examined at the end of the menstrual cycle or during the following month.

Abnormal uterus

Myomas (fibroids)

Myomas appear in various ways on ultrasound examination. Most will be seen as multiple, well defined, homogeneous, hypoechogenic, nodular masses, either subserosal, submucosal or interstitial. Older myomas become hyperechogenic and some will develop a complex echo pattern as a result of central necrosis. There may be bright echoes from calcification. Rapidly growing myomas, as may occur in pregnancy, may simulate hypoechogenic cysts. Multiple projections are needed to differentiate between myomas and tubo-ovarian masses. Some myomas are pedunculated. Uterine myomas can indent the posterior wall of the bladder (Fig. 146).

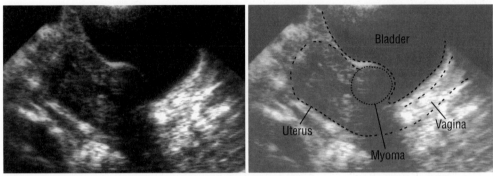

Fig. 146a. Longitudinal scan: a uterine myoma elevating the posterior wall of the bladder.

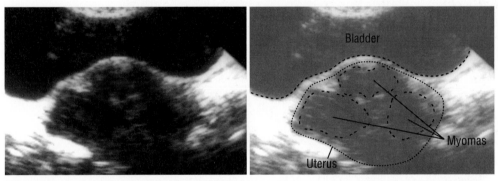

Fig. 146b. Transverse scan: a uterus enlarged by multiple myomas, which distort the bladder.

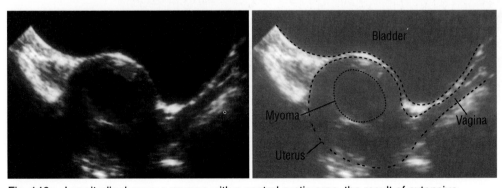

Fig. 146c. Longitudinal scan: a myoma with a central cystic area, the result of extensive necrosis.

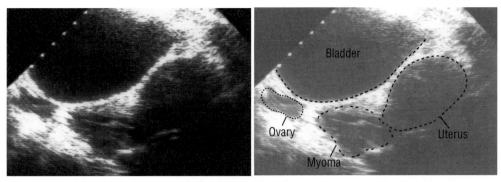

Fig. 146d. Pedunculated myoma shown as an irregular complex mass, lying between the ovary and the uterus.

Myomas may also contain calcium, which can present as hyperechogenic structures with distal shadowing (Fig. 146e). Myomas are almost always multiple (Fig. 146b) and frequently distort the normal contours and the endometrial canal of the uterus.

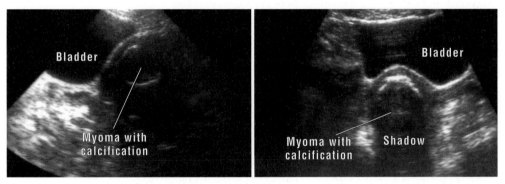

Fig. 146e. Longitudinal (left) and transverse (right) scans: a uterine myoma with peripheral calcification.

Myomas can also originate in the cervical part of the uterus and may cause distortion or blockage of the cervical canal (Fig. 146f).

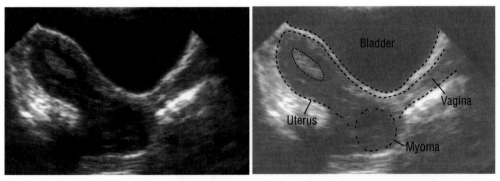

Fig. 146f. Longitudinal scan: a myoma distorting the posterior part of the uterine cervix.

Developmental variants

A bicornuate uterus may be identified by the presence of two endometrial canals or two uterine fundi on transverse scans (Fig. 147). Care must be taken not to confuse a bicornuate uterus with an adnexal mass. A double uterus has two endometrial canals and two cervices: if there is an adnexal or other mass, there will be only one canal.

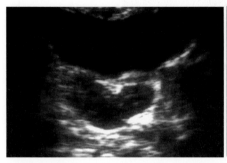 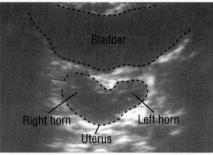

Fig. 147a. Transverse scan: a bicornuate uterus.

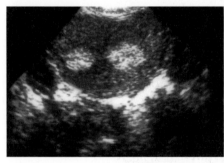 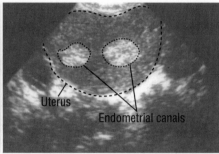

Fig. 147b. Transverse scan: a bicornuate uterus; there are two distinct endometrial canals.

The endometrium (lining of the uterus)

The normal pattern varies with the stage of the menstrual cycle. In the secretory phase (at the beginning of the cycle) the endometrium appears thin and hypoechogenic. In the proliferative phase (mid-cycle) the central part of the endometrium becomes hyperechogenic and is surrounded by a hypoechogenic rim. During the menstrual phase the endometrial cavity becomes totally hyperechogenic and thickened owing to sloughing endometrial tissue and blood clots (Fig. 148) (see also pp. 198 and 199).

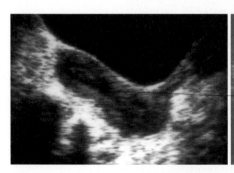 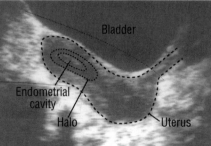

Fig. 148a. Longitudinal scan: the uterine endometrium at the proliferative mid-cycle phase.

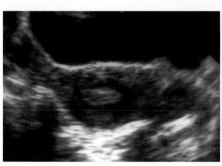 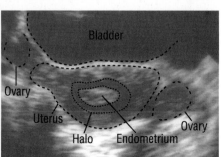

Fig. 148b. Transverse scan of the same patient at the same phase in the cycle.

In women with an imperforate hymen, or in those who have undergone ritual circumcision, blood may accumulate in the endometrial canal (haematometrium) or in the vagina (haematocolpos) and will be hypoechogenic compared with the endometrium (Fig. 149).

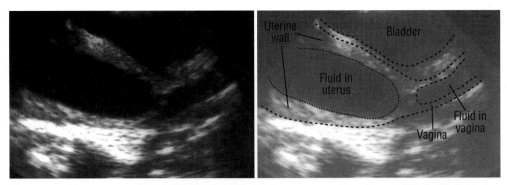

Fig. 149a. Haematometrium and haematocolpos: the uterus and vagina are filled with fluid because the hymen is imperforate.

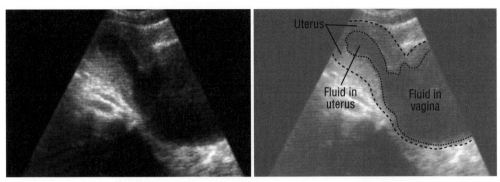

Fig. 149b. Haematometrium and haematocolpos: the uterine cavity and the vagina are filled with fluid.

The endometrial canal may be filled with pus from infection (pyometria). This will appear hypoechogenic with internal echoes (Fig. 149c). Fluid resulting from infection may also collect in the fallopian tubes (hydrosalpinx) and may spread to the cul-de-sac (Fig. 150) (see also p. 220).

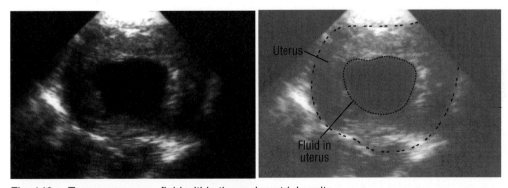

Fig. 149c. Transverse scan: fluid within the endometrial cavity.

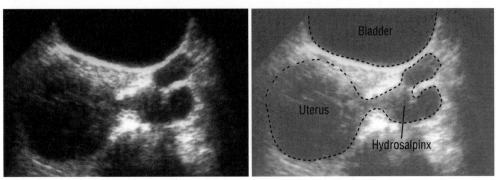

Fig. 150. Transverse scan: hydrosalpinx.

Malignant disease

A poorly defined mass within the uterus may be malignant and is usually an endometrial carcinoma. The endometrium becomes hyperplastic and the hypoechogenic tumour may spread into the myometrium. When the tumour is advanced, there may be necrosis, resulting in a complex ultrasound pattern: there may be distension of the endometrial cavity of the uterus (Fig. 151).

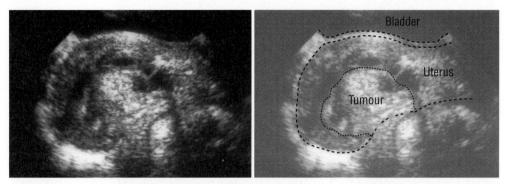

Fig. 151a. Longitudinal midline scan: a large endometrial carcinoma distends the cavity of the uterus and is invading the posterior myometrium.

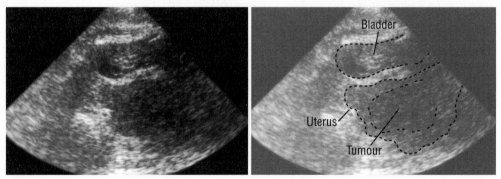

Fig. 151b. Longitudinal scan: an extensive endometrial carcinoma enlarging and distorting the uterus.

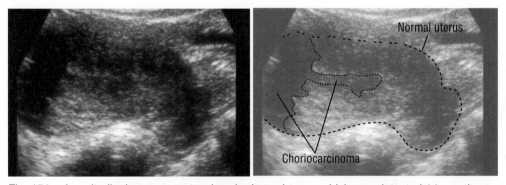

Fig. 151c. Longitudinal scan: an extensive choriocarcinoma, which was detected 14 months after a normal pregnancy and now distorts the uterus.

A small carcinoma of the cervix cannot always be recognized by ultrasound.

Early carcinoma of the cervix is very difficult to recognize with ultrasound. Any ill-defined mass in the cervix is likely to be malignant (most myomas are well defined and the bright echoes of calcification may be seen). If the tumour is large, the echo pattern will be complex and very varied (Fig. 152). The tumour may infiltrate the surrounding tissues, and the bladder, vagina and rectum should be carefully scanned (see p. 207 for the use of fluid to obtain better definition).

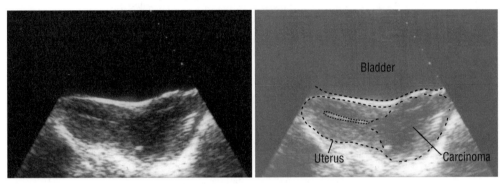

Fig. 152. Longitudinal scan: a large carcinoma of the cervix uteri.

Uterine endometriosis

Hypoechogenic spaces in the myometrium near the endometrium may represent adenomyosis (uterine endometriosis). The spaces will be more prominent during and immediately after menstruation. Small retention cysts (follicles) in the uterine cervix, close to the canal, should not be mistaken for endometriosis. A pelvic mass may be an endometrioma (Fig. 153) (see also Fig. 159, p. 219) or ectopic pregnancy (p. 222).

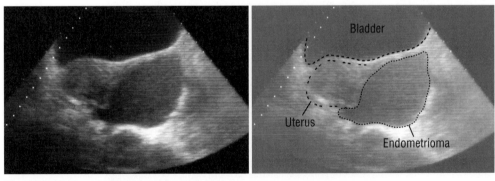

Fig. 153. Transverse scan: endometrioma.

Remember: always vary the gain setting throughout pelvic ultrasound examinations to obtain the best images.

Abnormal ovary

The normal ovary is slightly less echogenic than the uterus and less homogeneous because of the presence of small follicles (Fig. 154) (see also pp. 208–209). Identification in postmenopausal women can be difficult, particularly after the age of 50 (see pp. 204–207).

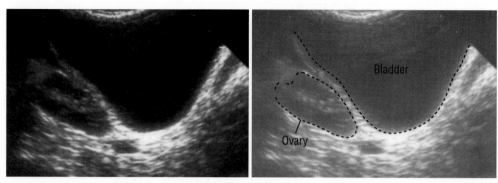

Fig. 154. Longitudinal scan: a normal ovary.

Ovarian cysts

A follicle is a physiological ovarian cyst which normally disappears during the second half of the menstrual cycle (see p. 209). If the follicle fails to rupture in mid-cycle, it will become a follicular cyst, which is one cause of ovarian cysts; these may be over 3 cm in diameter. Immediately after rupture there may be a little fluid in the cul-de-sac (Fig. 138, p. 201).

A simple cyst has smooth walls, no internal echoes, good distal wall enhancement and is almost always benign (Fig. 155a). Vestigial embryonic structures in the pelvis can give rise to simple cysts.

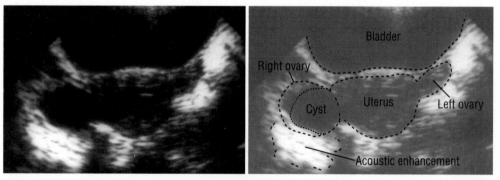

Fig. 155a. Transverse scan: an ovarian cyst with smooth walls.

On ultrasound, ovarian cysts can appear cystic or almost solid or complex with internal echoes from haemorrhage, nodules or septations. Complex cysts have strong back wall enhancement and variable internal patterns and are more likely to be malignant.

Small or medium-sized ovarian cysts lying behind the uterus or bladder cannot be seen easily, particularly if the bladder is only partly filled. Large ovarian cysts often lie above the uterine fundus when the bladder is full, and may cause distortion of the bladder by external pressure (Fig. 155b). A very large cystic mass may be mistaken for the urinary bladder: both should be identified (Fig. 155c) (see also pp. 204–207 for useful scanning techniques).

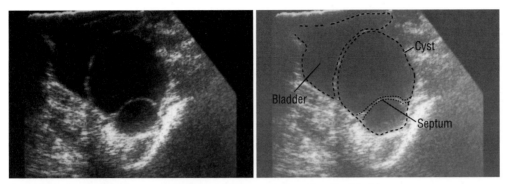

Fig. 155b. Longitudinal scan: a septate ovarian cyst distorting the bladder.

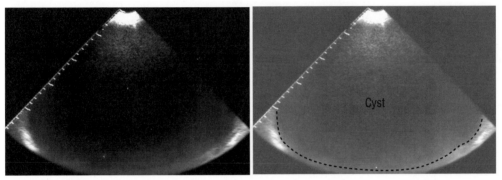

Fig. 155c. Longitudinal scan: an ovarian cyst which is so large that it may be mistaken for the urinary bladder.

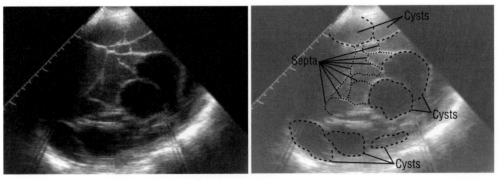

Fig. 155d. A multiseptate ovarian cyst.

Dermoid cysts (cystic teratomas) appear as solid or complex masses with areas of acoustic shadowing due to calcification in bone or teeth. If there is any doubt, X-ray the pelvis (Fig. 156).

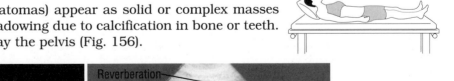

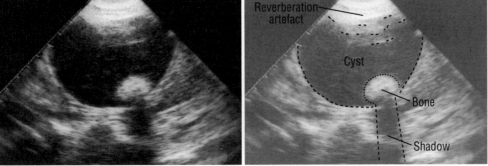

Fig. 156. A dermoid cyst with internal bone, which is causing acoustic shadowing.

Pelvic echinococcal (hydatid) cysts

Hydatid cysts are of different sizes, often multiple and in almost any position; some have internal septa (Fig. 157). If echinococcosis is suspected, scan the liver and X-ray the chest for other cysts.

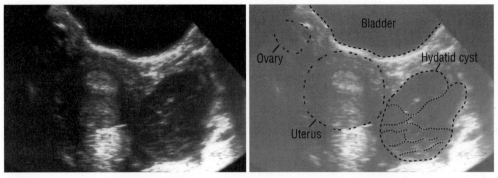

Fig. 157a. Transverse scan: an echinococcal (hydatid) cyst with internal septa.

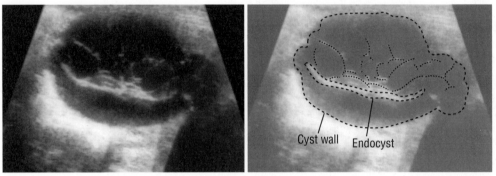

Fig. 157b. An enlarged view of the same hydatid cyst from a different angle; there is separation of the endocyst (the germinal membrane) from the external cyst wall.

Solid ovarian masses

Solid masses are rare and have often undergone necrosis or internal haemorrhage by the time they can be recognized ultrasonically. Solid ovarian masses may be confused with pedunculated fibroids and a careful search for a uterine connection should be made (Fig. 158).

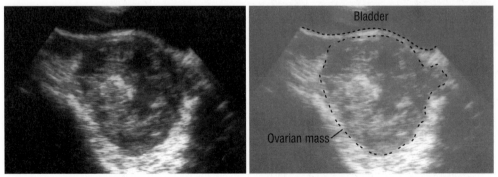

Fig. 158. Transverse scan: a large, solid, non-homogeneous ovarian mass elevating the posterior wall of the bladder.

Cystic masses in the pelvis of postmenopausal women are probably malignant.

Pelvic inflammatory disease

In pelvic inflammatory disease, there may be adhesions, distortion of the tissues, displacement of the uterus or ovaries, fixation, and changes in the echogenicity of the parametrial tissues. However, ultrasound may be normal and clinical examination may be more accurate. Pelvic tuberculosis cannot be distinguished from other inflammatory processes. A mass may be an endometrioma (Fig. 159), abscess or ectopic pregnancy; exact localization may be difficult less (see also pp.220 and 222).

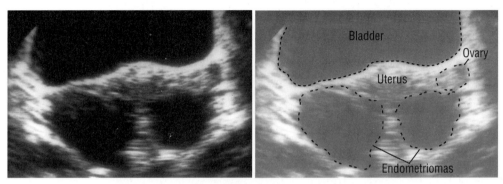

Fig. 159. Transverse scan: bilateral, predominantly cystic, endometriomas.

Fluid in the pelvis (ascites)

If there is excess fluid, suspect ascites, blood, pus or the contents of a ruptured cyst. Multiple projections will help assessment (Fig. 160).

The fluid may be echo-free or produce internal echoes as a result of debris. Fluid collections may also be found in the vagina and in the endometrial canal (p. 213) (see p. 201 for normal pelvic fluid).

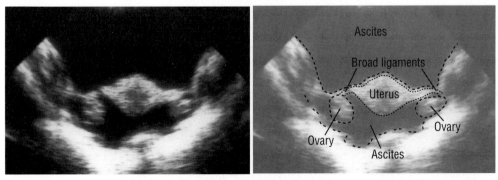

Fig. 160a. Longitudinal scan: the uterus appears to be floating in peritoneal fluid (ascites).

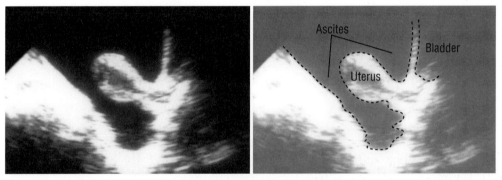

Fig. 160b. Transverse scan: the same patient. The ovaries also seem to be floating.

There are many causes of pelvic masses. Ultrasound cannot always distinguish between them.

Pelvic abscess

Any localized, complex pelvic mass may be inflammatory, but pyogenic and tuberculous infections look the same. It is often impossible to be sure of the exact location or etiology of an inflammatory mass: clinical examination is very important (Fig. 161).

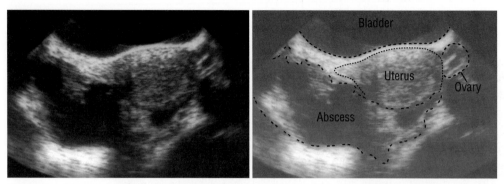

Fig. 161a. Transverse scan: a pelvic abscess shown as an irregular complex mass.

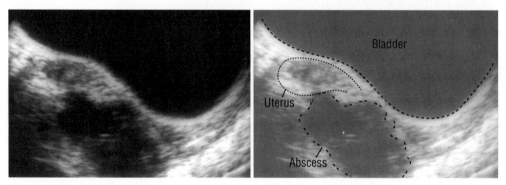

Fig. 161b. Longitudinal scan: the same pelvic abscess lying partly behind the uterus.

Fallopian tubes

It is not easy to demonstrate a normal fallopian tube with ultrasound. The fallopian tubes vary in both size and position, and it is difficult to be sure that there is an abnormality unless there is a significant local change, for example, partial enlargement of one tube. If the tubes are fluid-filled, it may be difficult to differentiate bowel, but bowel shows peristalsis whereas the fallopian tubes will not alter significantly over a period of a few hours. Tubal obstruction cannot be recognized with ultrasound unless there is tubal swelling above it.

Enlargement of part of one fallopian tube may be due to an ectopic pregnancy (see p. 222) which will cause a tubular, fluid-filled, echo-free (or mixed) mass near to the uterus. However, any pyosalpinx (tuberculous or pyogenic) will appear very similar. Clinical signs are the only way to differentiate a hydrosalpinx from a pyosalpinx (Fig. 162).

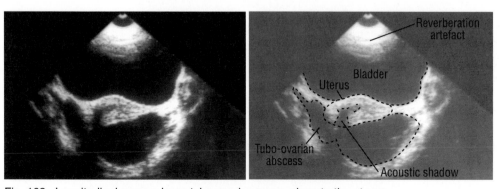

Fig. 162. Longitudinal scan: a large tubo-ovarian mass, close to the uterus.

Pelvic varices

Dilated pelvic veins can be painful, particularly in the premenstrual phase. Ultrasound will demonstrate multiple echo-free, tubular structures around the uterus and occasionally between the uterus and the bladder. There may be only a single dilated vein, which may be mistaken for a hydrosalpinx. Differentiation can be made by examining the patient tilted head downwards. A dilated vein will empty in this position, whereas a hydrosalpinx will not change (Fig. 163).

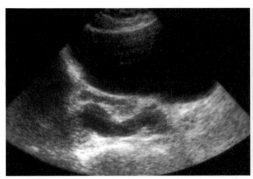 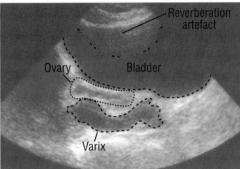

Fig. 163. Longitudinal scan of a patient with pelvic varices.

There are many causes of pelvic masses. Ultrasound cannot always distinguish between them. Remember also:

- **A large pelvic mass may compress the ureter resulting in hydronephrosis. If a pelvic mass is identified, the kidneys should be evaluated to rule out hydronephrosis (pp. 160–161).**

- **Masses in the bowel (e.g. inflammatory or parasitic) may be confused with a pelvic mass. Watch for peristalsis (pp. 143–144).**

- **A cleansing enema may be used to remove faecal material from the colon, or to insert fluid into the rectum (p. 207) to clarify pelvic anatomy.**

Ectopic pregnancy

A pelvic mass in a woman of childbearing age may be an ectopic pregnancy. Although ultrasound may be useful, it is not an entirely reliable method of diagnosing ectopic pregnancy. It is sometimes possible to demonstrate the ectopic sac and an embryo (see p. 230), but more commonly there is pooled blood in the pelvic cul-de-sac and an enlarged fluid-filled fallopian tube (Fig. 164) (see also p. 220).

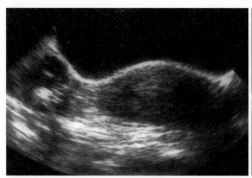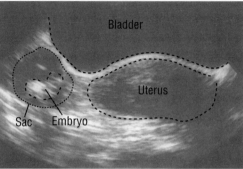

Fig. 164a. Transverse scan of an ectopic pregnancy, showing a small embryo. Movement of the embryo's heart could be seen.

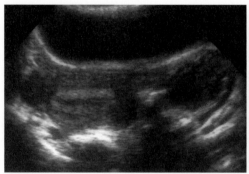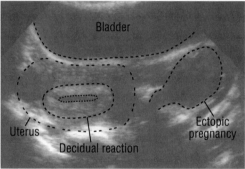

Fig. 164b. Transverse scan: ectopic pregnancy causing a decidual reaction in the uterus due to endocrine stimulation. The pregnancy lies in the left adnexa.

Be careful.

- A normal transabdominal pelvic ultrasound examination does *not* exclude ectopic pregnancy.

- With a reliable positive pregnancy test, a normal ultrasound examination strongly suggests ectopic pregnancy.

- Even when an intrauterine pregnancy *is* demonstrated, there may be a co-existing ectopic pregnancy.

- Careful correlation with the clinical history and with the clinical examination is essential.

CHAPTER 17

Obstetrics

Introduction

Diagnostic ultrasound has been used in obstetrics for nearly 30 years. Although generally considered safe, there is continuing study and research to confirm this. It is a very important technique for examining pregnant women and can be used when clinically indicated at any time during pregnancy.

Is ultrasound safe during pregnancy?

Yes, as far as is known. However, it should be used only when there is a good clinical reason.

Is a clinically normal pregnancy a good reason for using ultrasound?

This is controversial and is still being investigated. However, there is agreement that there are two stages during a normal pregnancy when ultrasound scans will be the most useful and provide the most information.

These stages are:

1. At **18–22 weeks** after the first day of the woman's last menstrual period
2. At **32–36 weeks** after the first day of the woman's last menstrual period

Most informative times for a first scan

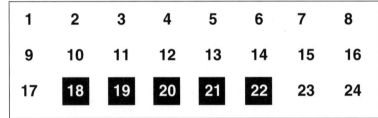

weeks

Most informative times for a second scan

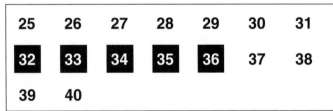

weeks

When is ultrasound not recommended?

There is no indication for an ultrasound examination in the first trimester of pregnancy unless there is a clinical abnormality (see p. 226).

Why is a scan not recommended at the mother's first visit?

Some physicians **do** recommend an ultrasound examination at the time of the mother's first visit, but there is no reason to do this provided the clinical examination is normal. When considered necessary, scanning during weeks 18–22 of pregnancy will provide much more important information.

There is no need to perform ultrasound every month or during every antenatal visit, unless there is a clinical reason to suspect an abnormality that needs to be investigated further.

Why consider scanning during a normal pregnancy?

Many physicians consider that scanning is unnecessary during a clinically normal pregnancy. Others recommend scanning because many obstetric abnormalities cannot be detected by clinical examination.

1. 90% of developmental fetal abnormalities occur without any family history and very few of the mothers show any obvious risk factors.

2. There can be significant fetal abnormalities even in a clinically normal pregnancy.

3. Neither clinical examination nor a family history is an entirely reliable way to detect multiple pregnancy.

4. A significant number of mothers with a low-lying placenta (placenta praevla) show no evidence until bleeding starts at the onset of labour. The situation can then be extremely dangerous, especially if the patient is a long way from the nearest hospital.

5. Up to 50% of mothers who claim to know their obstetric dates with certainty are in fact more than two weeks in error when gestational age is calculated with ultrasound. A discrepancy of two weeks can be critical for the survival of an infant who has to be delivered early because of some antenatal complication.

What are the objections to scanning during a normal pregnancy?

Many physicians believe that the possible risks and the costs of scanning every clinically normal pregnancy are not justified by the benefits for the patient.

This decision, to scan or not to scan a normal pregnancy, must be made by the physician and each patient. There are no universally accepted guidelines at present.

The determination of the sex of the fetus is not a valid indication for ultrasound except when there is a strong familial risk of a sex-linked genetic disorder.

What is important in the 18–22 week scan?

This is the best time during pregnancy to:

1. establish the gestational age accurately;
2. diagnose multiple pregnancy;
3. diagnose fetal abnormalities;
4. locate the placenta and identify patients in whom there is a risk of placenta praevia;
5. recognize myomas or any other unexpected pelvic mass that may interfere with pregnancy or delivery.

What is important in the 32–36 week scan?

This is the best time during pregnancy to:

1. recognize intrauterine growth retardation;
2. recognize fetal anomalies that were not detected at the first scan;
3. confirm the presentation and position of the fetus;
4. locate the placenta accurately;
5. assess the amount of amniotic fluid;
6. exclude possible complications, e.g. myoma, ovarian tumour.

What are the indications for a scan before 18 weeks?

The patient should have a careful clinical examination as soon as there is either a positive pregnancy test or a missed menstrual period. An ultrasound scan is helpful when there is clinical evidence that the pregnancy may not be normal or if there is any doubt about the gestational age.

What can be learned from an early scan (before 18 weeks)?

Ultrasound in the early weeks of pregnancy can:

1. confirm the pregnancy;
2. accurately estimate gestational age;
3. locate the pregnancy (intra- or extrauterine);
4. recognize single or multiple pregnancy;
5. exclude molar pregnancy;
6. exclude pseudo-pregnancy due to a pelvic mass or hormone-secreting ovarian tumour;
7. diagnose myomas or ovarian masses which might interfere with normal delivery.

Preparation

1. **Preparation of the patient**. The bladder must be full. Give 4 or 5 glasses of fluid and examine after one hour (do not allow the patient to micturate). Alternatively, fill the bladder through a urethral catheter with sterile normal saline: stop when the patient feels uncomfortable. Avoid catheterization if possible because of the risk of infection.

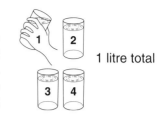

1 litre total

2. **Position of the patient**. The patient is usually scanned while lying comfortably on her back (supine). It may be necessary to rotate the patient after the preliminary scans.

   Apply coupling agent liberally to the lower abdomen: it is not usually necessary to cover the pubic hair but, if required, apply freely.

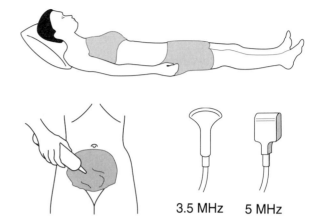

3. **Choice of transducer**. Use a 3.5 MHz transducer. Use a 5 MHz transducer for thin women.

3.5 MHz   5 MHz

4. **Setting the correct gain**. Position the transducer longitudinally over the full bladder and adjust the gain to produce the best image.

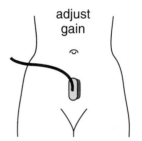

adjust gain

Early pregnancy

Location of the gestational sac is the first evidence of pregnancy. It can often be recognized in the uterus after five weeks of amenorrhoea, and may be located asymmetrically (Fig. 165).

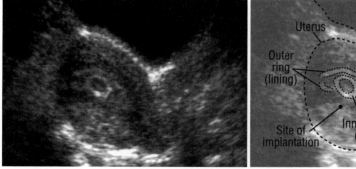
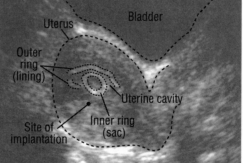

Fig. 165. The gestational sac at 5–6 weeks. The centre is hypoechogenic, surrounded by a double echogenic ring. The inner ring is complete and is the gestational sac. The outer ring is incomplete and is the lining of the uterus. These two rings are separated by the anechogenic space of the residual endometrial (uterine) cavity.

All normal pregnancies should be recognizable after 6 weeks as a well defined "double echogenic ring" in the uterus. The inner ring is of uniform echogenicity and is 2 mm or more thick. Around it is a thin echogenic ring, which does not encircle the entire gestational sac. Between the two rings is the anechogenic residual uterine cavity (Fig. 165, p. 227).

At 5–6 weeks, the greatest diameter of the gestational sac is approximately 1–2 cm. At 8 weeks the sac should occupy half the uterus; at 9 weeks it should take up two-thirds of the uterus, and at 10 weeks it should fill the uterus.

The gestational age can be estimated to within one week from the mean dimension of the sac. Using a longitudinal scan, measure the maximum dimensions of the sac in the long axis (length), and at 90° to this in the antero–posterior (AP) dimension (Fig. 166, upper scan). Make a transverse scan at right angles to the longitudinal scan plane and measure the greatest width of the sac (Fig. 166, lower scan). The mean dimension of the sac is the sum of these three measurements divided by 3.

$$\text{Mean gestational sac dimension} = \frac{\text{Length} + \text{AP} + \text{Width}}{3}$$

The gestational age of the fetus can be estimated by reference to local standard development tables (see also p. 236).

> **Five or six weeks is the earliest stage at which a pregnancy can be recognized with ultrasound.**

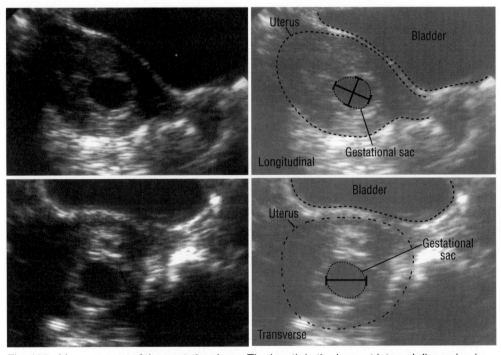

Fig. 166. Measurement of the gestational sac. The length is the longest internal dimension in the longitudinal plane (upper). The antero–posterior measurement is the widest part of the sac at right angles to the length (upper). The width is the widest part in a transverse scan (lower).

Intrauterine contraceptive device (IUD)

Is the IUD there?

Ultrasound is an ideal way to determine whether an intrauterine contraceptive device is in the uterus in its correct position, or whether it has moved outside the uterus (see also p. 201).

If the patient believes that there is an intrauterine device but it cannot be imaged within the uterus or pelvis, the whole abdomen should be scanned. IUDs can migrate as far as the splenic area. If there is still any doubt, a plain X-ray of the abdomen should be taken (provided pregnancy has been excluded), making sure that it includes the whole abdomen from the diaphragm to the bottom of the pelvis.

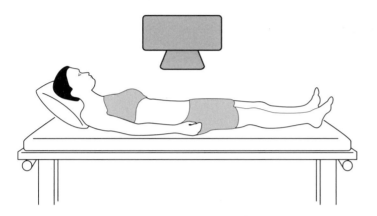

IUD and normal pregnancy

If the IUD is located well away from the implantation site of the embryo, pregnancy can be allowed to progress without interference (Fig. 167).

If the IUD is partially expelled, the pregnancy can be allowed to progress without interference.

If the IUD strings can be seen in the vagina, the device can be carefully removed.

In all other cases, spontaneous abortion is likely to occur and the patient should be warned of this possibility.

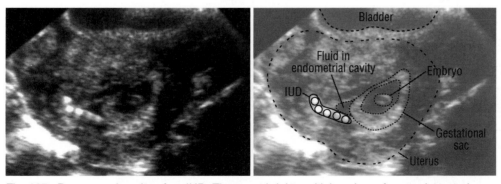

Fig. 167. Pregnancy in spite of an IUD. There are bright multiple echoes from an intrauterine loop next to the gestational sac.

Ectopic pregnancy

If there is an ectopic pregnancy, a gestational sac may be seen outside the uterus. Sometimes there is a sac-like structure in the uterus despite the pregnancy being ectopic (Fig. 168). The real sac can be distinguished from the "pseudosac" by the presence of fetal parts, a yolk sac within the real sac or by a single ring around the pseudosac instead of a double ring (see p. 228) (see also p. 222).

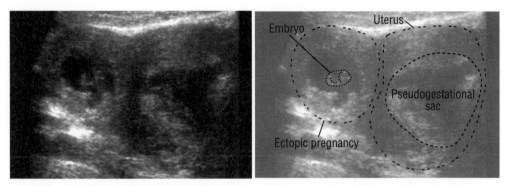

Fig. 168. An embryo within an extrauterine mass. There is a well-defined sac in the uterus, containing fluid only.

The embryo

Although the gestational sac can be recognized at 5 weeks in some patients and at 6 weeks in the majority, the embryo does not become visible until the eighth gestational week (Fig. 169a). It will then be shown as a focal area of echoes, often lying eccentrically within the gestational sac. If the fetus is alive, the heart will be recognized lying in mid-embryo, usually seeming to lie anterior to the rest of the thorax.

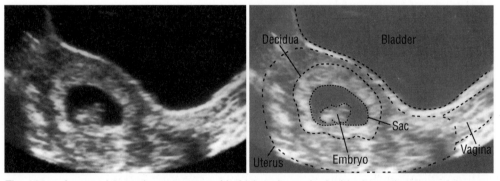

Fig. 169a. A normal 9-week pregnancy, with thick, echogenic decidual reaction around the sac.

After the ninth or tenth week, the fetal head can be distinguished from the body and movements can be seen. At 10 weeks the fetus becomes more human in appearance (Fig. 169b). After the twelfth week, the skull becomes visible.

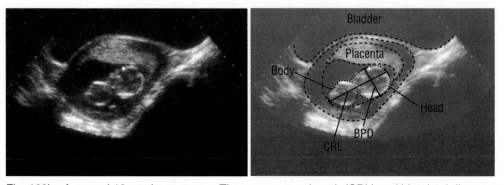

Fig. 169b. A normal 12-week pregnancy. The crown–rump length (CRL) and biparietal diameter (BPD) are shown (see pp. 236–237).

The yolk sac

From about 7 weeks onwards, it is usually possible to see a round cystic structure about 4–5 mm in diameter adjacent to the fetus. This is the yolk sac, the site of the earliest blood cell formation. It disappears at about the eleventh week. The yolk sac may not be seen in all pregnancies, even when quite normal.

It is important to recognize that this cystic shadow is the yolk sac and *not* mistake it for a second, twin embryo (Fig. 170). (The yolk sac is not included in crown–rump measurements.)

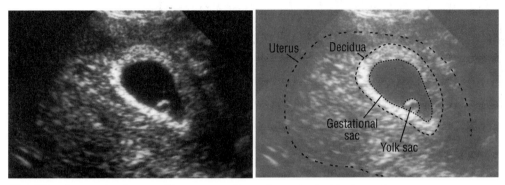

Fig. 170. A normal yolk sac with a surrounding echogenic decidual reaction.

Multiple pregnancy

The earliest it is possible to diagnose multiple pregnancy is at about 8 weeks' gestation; however, not all gestational sacs go on to contain a viable fetus. *Never* tell a patient that she has a multiple pregnancy until more than one viable fetus is recognized and each is growing normally. This is usually after about 14 weeks, and is best seen between 18 and 22 weeks (Fig. 171).

Multiple pregnancy can usually be recognized at about 8 weeks, but do not tell the patient until confirmed by a scan after 14 weeks.

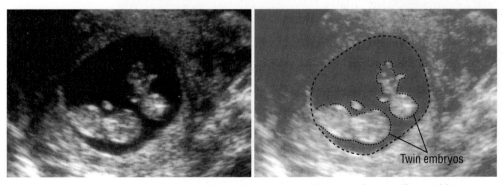

Fig. 171. Twin pregnancy: each embryo must be measured separately, usually requiring scans at different angles.

If a multiple pregnancy is suspected in early pregnancy, use a sagittal scan. The abdominal muscles may produce a misleading artefact (the lens effect, p. 36).

Abnormalities in the first three months of pregnancy

Small gestational sac

A small gestational sac is usually due to a blighted ovum (anembryonic gestation) and is a fairly common finding. On ultrasound examination the gestational sac is found to be smaller than expected for the gestational age, and the fetus cannot be demonstrated (Fig. 172).

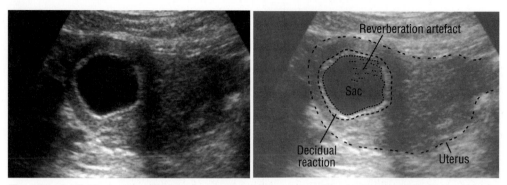

Fig. 172. A blighted ovum. The sac is round, but the surrounding decidua is irregular and there is no embryo.

If an early pregnancy is clinically normal, but an ultrasound scan shows an enlarged uterus, an anembryonic gestation should be suspected: repeat the examination after 7 days. If the pregnancy is normal, the sac should have grown, and the fetus and the heart activity should be clearly seen at the second examination.

Fetal death (spontaneous abortion)

When there is a fetal or embryonic death, the patient may remain clinically normal and may continue to feel pregnant for days. There may be a history of bleeding or abdominal cramp. The uterus may be normal, small, or even enlarged if there is significant intrauterine haematoma. The fetal pole may be visible but no heart action will be demonstrated. If the examination is made during the first 8 weeks of pregnancy, it should be repeated after another 7 days. After the eighth week, fetal life should always be demonstrable in a normal pregnancy (Fig. 173).

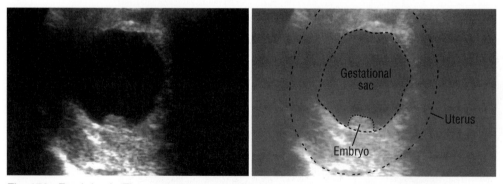

Fig. 173. Fetal death. The sac is the correct size for the expected gestational age, but the embryo is too small (and no heart beat was seen).

It should always be possible to demonstrate fetal heart activity after the eighth week of pregnancy.

Empty uterus

The patient will have a history of amenorrhoea followed by loss of blood, sometimes with recognition of the fetus. If this is recent, the uterus may still be large, approximately the expected size for gestational age. The scan will show the uterus to be empty.

Incomplete abortion

The patient may have a history of amenorrhoea, followed by loss of blood; she may have seen the fetus. If this is recent, the uterus may still be large, approximately the expected size for gestational age. However, the uterus may be empty and the endometrial canal may be normal. If the abortion is incomplete, the uterus will be smaller than expected for gestational age and filled with an abnormally shaped sac (Fig. 174) or with an amorphous mass of variable size, shape and echogenicity. This is the retained placenta and blood clots (see also p. 235). There will be no sign of fetal life.

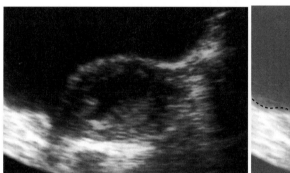
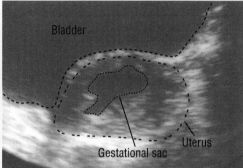

Fig. 174. An incomplete abortion. The uterus is bulky, the sac is irregular and poorly echogenic. There is no embryo.

It can be difficult to recognize the retained products of conception after a spontaneous abortion. This diagnosis should not be made unless there are identifiable parts, such a yolk sac, gestational sac or dead embryo. Endometrial thickening is not a reliable way of recognizing or excluding retained products of conception, and a molar pregnancy must be excluded (Fig. 175).

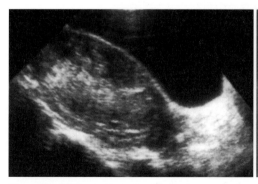
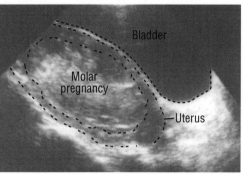

Fig. 175. Molar pregnancy. There is no sac, and the uterus is filled with echogenic material without any retained products of conception.

Be warned: the patient's estimate of gestational age is not always accurate.

Large uterus

The commonest causes of a uterus larger than expected are:

- Hydatidiform mole.
- Choriocarcinoma.
- Intrauterine bleeding associated with spontaneous abortion.
- Uterine myoma (fibroids).

1. **Hydatidiform mole**. Clinical findings are nonspecific. Ultrasound is almost always abnormal and shows a large uterus filled with a mass of uniform echoes providing a regular speckled appearance: the "snow-storm" effect. It may be difficult to distinguish a mole from echogenic blood within the uterus, but blood is usually more heterogeneous and less echogenic than a mole, which may have cystic spaces (vesicles). In older patients in particular, a large myoma may cause confusion, but moles will have stronger back wall echoes and central necrosis (Fig. 176). It is important to remember that the fetus may still be present and only part of the placenta may be affected. Embryos in association with moles have a high incidence of chromosomal abnormalities.

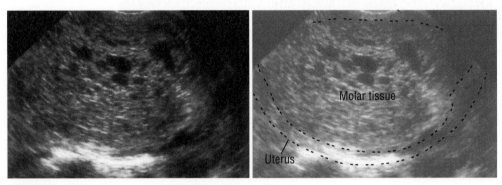

Fig. 176a. A hydatidiform mole filling the uterus with echogenic and cystic tissue.

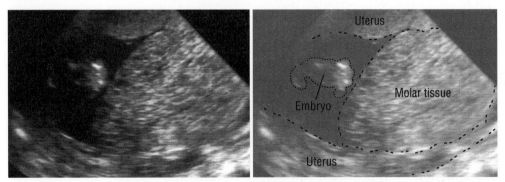

Fig. 176b. A hydatidiform mole with a living embryo. There is an increased risk of chromosomal abnormalities in the fetus and, as pregnancy progresses, there is an increasing likelihood of fetal death.

2. **Choriocarcinoma** may be indistinguishable from a hydatidiform mole by ultrasound, but it should be considered if the uterus is much larger than expected and the ultrasound scan shows areas of haemorrhage and necrosis rather than the uniform echoes of a mole. The pattern of choriocarcinoma may be mixed, with both solid and fluid echoes, rather than the homogeneous snow-storm effect of a mole. Rarely there may be disease elsewhere: X-ray the chest to exclude metastases.

3. **Intrauterine haemorrhage due to threatened or spontaneous abortion**. This is mainly a clinical diagnosis based on bleeding in early pregnancy: ultrasound may show a varying amount of blood in the uterus, separating the chorioamniotic membrane from the decidua (the lining of the membrane of the uterus), which shows as a clearly defined anechogenic area. The blood may be completely anechogenic or echogenic. It is usually heterogeneous (Fig. 177). It is very important to search for signs of fetal life because this will influence the way the patient is managed. If there is any doubt, repeat scans at one- or two-week intervals to evaluate the progress of the pregnancy.

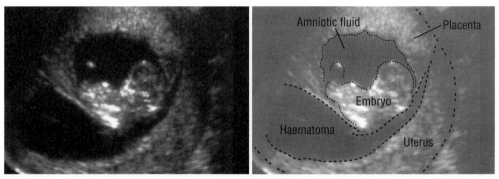

Fig. 177. A poorly echogenic intrauterine haematoma, which is lifting the edge of the placenta and distorting the gestational sac. This haematoma was absorbed and the embryo survived.

> **If there is any doubt after one scan, repeat in one or two weeks.**

4. **Large irregular uterus**. In the first trimester a large, irregular uterus is usually due to uterine myomas (Fig. 178). Record the size and position of the myomas and estimate the potential difficulties that they may cause during labour. The myomas should be reviewed at 32–36 weeks' gestation. The central area may become necrotic, showing a mixed or echo-free pattern. This does not necessarily have any clinical significance. A myoma can be mimicked by contraction of the uterine muscle, and the scan should be repeated after 20–30 minutes to see if the contraction area changes. Contractions are normal and indent the inner aspect of the uterus (see p. 273).

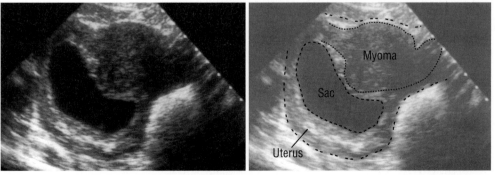

Fig. 178. A myoma pressing on the gestational sac and also bulging outward from the uterus. There is varying echogenicity in the myoma.

Estimation of fetal size and age (fetal biometry)

If gestational age and fetal development are to be estimated, measurements must be obtained and then compared with local standard values. Although there are many alternative measurements that can be made, only a few are accurate and reliable.

Crown–rump length measurement (CRL)

The crown–rump length is the most reliable parameter for estimating gestational age up to the eleventh week. After that, the curvature of the fetus affects the reliability of the measurement. From the twelfth week onwards, the biparietal diameter is more accurate.

There is excellent correlation between the crown–rump length and gestational age from the seventh to the eleventh week of pregnancy: biological variability is minimal and growth is not affected by pathological disorders.

Using scans in different directions, the longest length of the embryo should be found and a measurement made from the head (the cephalic pole) to the outer edge of the rump (Fig. 179). The yolk sac should not be included.

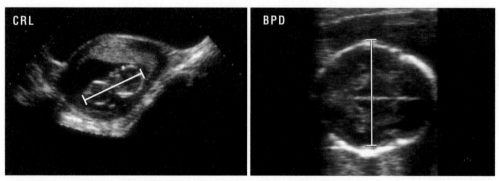

Fig. 179. Up to 11 weeks (left) measure the crown–rump length; after 11 weeks (right) measure the biparietal diameter.

Using scans in different directions, measure the fetus from head to buttock. Measure the longest length, ignoring any curvature.

Do not include the fetal limbs or the yolk sac in this measurement.

The gestational age can be determined from crown–rump length to within approximately one week using biometric tables. Make sure that you use tables that are appropriate for your patients and not derived from some quite different population.

Biparietal diameter

This is the most reliable method of estimating gestational age between the 12th and the 26th weeks. After that, its accuracy may be lessened by pathological disorders and biological variations that affect fetal growth. It must be considered together with other measurements, such as femoral length and abdominal circumference (Fig. 180).

The biparietal diameter (BPD) is the distance between the parietal eminences on either side of the skull and is, therefore, the widest diameter of the skull from side to side. Using scans at different angles, the transverse section will be recognized when the shape of the fetal skull is ovoid and the midline echo from the falx cerebri is interrupted by the cavum septi pellucidi and the thalami (see pp. 247–248). When this plane is found, the gain on the ultrasound unit should be reduced and measurements made from the outer table of the proximal skull (the part nearest to the transducer) to the inner table of the distal skull (the part farthest away from the transducer). The soft tissues over the skull are not included. This is the "leading-edge-to-leading-edge" technique.

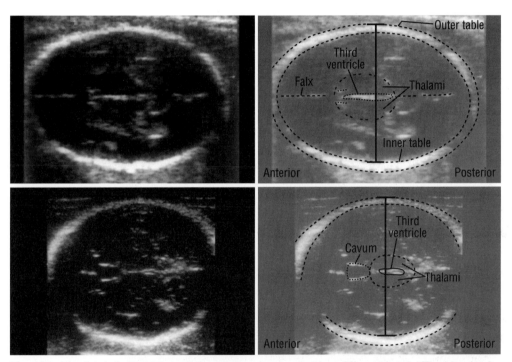

Fig. 180. The fetal skull at 24 weeks' gestation, scanned at two different levels. The biparietal diameter is the widest distance from the outer edge of the proximal skull to the inner edge of the distal skull. At the correct level the midline falx is interrupted by the cavum septi pellucidi.

Be careful.

If your ultrasound unit has a programmed comparative scale relating normal growth to the biparietal diameter, check the manual. Some older units base the scale on measurements made from the outside of the skull: others use measurements from the inside of the skull.

Whichever method you use, make sure the data are appropriate for your patients and not derived from a quite different population.

Fronto-occipital diameter

The fronto-occipital diameter is measured along the longest axis of the skull at the level of the biparietal diameter (BPD), from outer edge to outer edge.

Cephalic index

The BPD is a reliable estimate of gestational age except when the shape of the head is abnormal or there is an abnormality of the intracranial contents (Fig. 207, pp. 262–263). The adequacy of the head shape is determined by comparing its short axis to its long axis—the cephalic index.

$$\text{Cephalic index} \ = \ \frac{\text{Biparietal diameter}}{\text{Fronto-occipital diameter}} \times 100$$

Normal range (± 2 standard deviations) = 70–86

Head circumference

If the cephalic index is within the normal range, the BPD is acceptable as an estimate of gestational age. If the cephalic index is outside this range (less than 70 or greater than 86), the measured BPD should not be used to determine the gestational age. Instead, the head circumference can be used. On some ultrasound machines, this may be measured directly. It can also be calculated (Fig. 181).

$$\text{Head circumference} =$$
$$(\text{Biparietal diameter} + \text{Fronto–occipital diameter}) \times 1.57$$

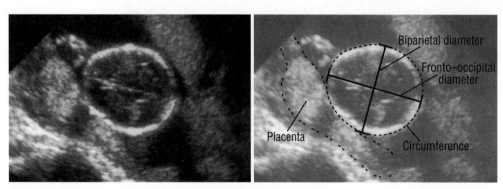

Fig. 181. The two ways of measuring the head circumference.

Abdominal circumference

Abdominal circumference is used to detect intrauterine growth disturbances. The measurement must be taken at the level of the fetal liver, which is very sensitive to deficient nutrition (Fig. 182a). If the measurement is less than normal there has probably been intrauterine growth retardation.

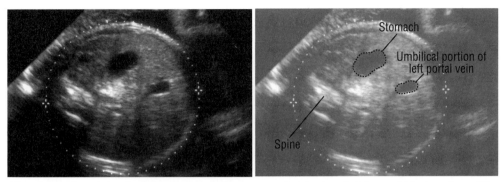

Fig. 182a. The abdominal circumference is measured at the level of the umbilical portion of the left portal vein. The diameters are measured from the skin surface.

It is most important that the scan shows a cross-section of the fetus that is as round as possible. Make sure that the correct level is being measured; look for the umbilical part of the left portal vein (see p. 256). The measurement must be made on a true transaxial plane, where the umbilical portion of the left portal vein enters and is entirely within the liver. The vein should be short, not elongated. If it is too long, the axis is too oblique (Fig. 182b).

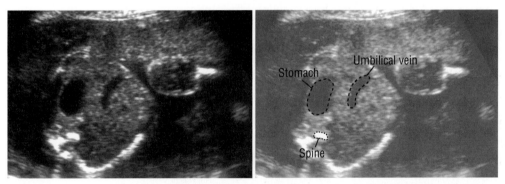

Fig. 182b. An incorrect angle to measure the abdominal circumference: the abdomen does not appear circular and the umbilical vein appears elongated.

When you have a scan at the correct level, measure the antero–posterior (AP) and transverse diameters. A medium gain setting should be used and the measurement must be from the outer edge of the fetal abdomen on one side to the outer edge on the other side. Calculate the abdominal circumference by multiplying the sum of the two measurements by 1.57.

Abdominal circumference =
(Antero-posterior diameter + Transverse diameter) × 1.57

If the abdominal circumference is less than the fifth percentile, it is small. If it is greater than the 95th percentile, it is large. (With some ultrasound units it is possible to make this measurement automatically by tracing the perimeter of the abdomen.)

Fetal long bone measurements

When measuring bone length, it is necessary to reduce the gain. It is usually easy to see fetal long bones from 13 weeks onwards. Find a projection that shows a transverse section of one of the long bones; then scan at 90° to this to obtain a longitudinal section. Measurements are made from one end of the bone to the other end (Fig. 183). The femur is the easiest bone to recognize and measure. If there is any doubt, also measure the limb on the other side.

The length of a bone, particularly the femoral length, can be used as a measure of gestational age when the head measurement is unreliable because of intracranial pathology. This occurs most frequently in the third trimester.

Bone length may also be compared with gestational age or biparietal diameter. A femoral or humeral measurement can be considered normal if it falls within two standard deviations of the mean for the known gestational age. It is proportional to the biparietal diameter if that measurement falls within two standard deviations of the mean biparietal diameter. A femur is short if it is more than two standard deviations below the mean. A skeletal dysplasia is likely only if the femur length is even smaller—5 mm smaller than two standard deviations below the mean.

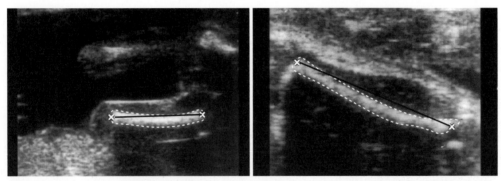

Fig. 183. The length of the femur is measured from end to end. In older fetuses (right), there is an ossification centre at the distal end of the femur; this is not included in the measurement.

There are limits to the accuracy of ultrasound:

- **Clinical and laboratory findings must be included in the assessment.**

- **When there is doubt, serial measurements should be made to assess the rate of embryonic and fetal growth at intervals of at least 2 weeks, or even 3 weeks.**

- **Do not scan at weekly intervals. The changes will be too slight for accurate assessment.**

Recognition of intrauterine growth retardation

The differentiation between *symmetrical* and *asymmetrical* growth retardation is important because they have different causes and different prognoses, and require different management.

1. **Symmetrical growth retardation—low-profile fetus**. In the low-profile fetus, (symmetrical) growth retardation is caused by a chromosomal abnormality, infection or maternal malnutrition, and becomes apparent earlier in gestation. The head:body ratio remains within normal limits and the fetus is symmetrically retarded: all the measurements are reduced in the same proportion.

2. **Asymmetrical growth retardation—late growth deceleration**. In late (asymmetrical) growth retardation, the fetal insults occur later in gestation (after the 32nd week) when fat accumulation should be greatest. The abdominal circumference will be significantly lower than normal and the head:body ratio will also be abnormal. Such growth retardation results from placental insufficiency in mothers with pre-eclampsia, oedema, proteinuria and hypertension. The prognosis for the fetus will be improved by adequate maternal treatment.

See pp. 242–244 for the required measurements and quality control.

Symmetrical growth retardation:

- Head:body ratio is normal.
- Starts in early pregnancy.
- All measurements reduced equally.

Asymmetrical growth retardation:

- Head:body ratio is abnormal.
- Starts in late pregnancy.
- Abdominal circumference is less than normal.

Ultrasound cannot always accurately diagnose intrauterine growth retardation.

Clinical and laboratory findings must be included in the assessment.

Measurements to assess fetal growth

A complete evaluation of fetal growth will require measurement of:

- the biparietal diameter (BPD);
- the head circumference;
- the abdominal circumference;
- the length of the femur.

What is the ultrasound-determined gestational age?

Comparison of fetal size and gestational age can provide a valuable indicator of intrauterine growth retardation. During the first routine scan, define the ultrasound gestational age based on the crown–rump length, head measurement and femur length. For follow-up studies, calculate age as the initial age (however derived) plus the number of weeks intervening.

> **At the first scan, estimated gestational age is based either on crown–rump length, or on head or femur measurement.**
>
> **At follow-up studies, gestational age is taken as the estimated age at the initial study plus the number of weeks intervening.**

Is the head size appropriate?

The head size (either biparietal diameter or head circumference) should be appropriate for the estimated ultrasound gestational age, i.e. the head measurement should fall within the range for the estimated gestational age.

Using the biparietal diameter alone, about 60% of growth-retarded fetuses will be detected. Using the abdominal circumference as well as other measurements, the sensitivity increases to 70–80%.

> **Tables used to estimate gestational age, fetal weight or development must be appropriate for the social group of the patient.**

Is the abdominal size appropriate?

Measure the abdomen and determine the appropriate percentile. An abdominal circumference less than the 5th percentile is abnormal and suggests intrauterine growth retardation.

What is the fetal weight? In what percentile does the weight fall?

Determine the fetal weight from biometric tables using at least two parameters and compare it with the standard distribution for the estimated gestational age. Intrauterine growth is considered to be retarded when the weight is lower than the 10th percentile. An abnormally low weight of the fetus is usually observed after the abdominal circumference and head:body ratio have become abnormal.

Is the head:body ratio normal, elevated or low?

The head:body ratio is calculated by dividing the head circumference by the abdominal circumference. It should be remembered that malformations may change the size of the head or abdomen. With normal anatomy, the head:body ratio can be considered normal if it lies between the 5th and 95th percentiles for the gestational age.

$$\text{Head:body ratio} = \frac{\text{Head circumference}}{\text{Abdominal circumference}}$$

The head:body ratio determines whether the growth retardation is symmetrical or asymmetrical. If the fetus is small and the ratio is normal, the fetus is symmetrically growth retarded. If the abdominal circumference or weight is low and the ratio is elevated (greater than the 95th percentile), there is asymmetrical growth retardation.

Asymmetrical growth retardation is easier to diagnose than symmetrical growth retardation.

> **When there is suspicion of intrauterine growth retardation, serial measurements should be made to assess the rate of fetal growth at intervals of at least two weeks, or even three weeks.**
>
> **Do not scan at weekly intervals. The changes will be too slight for accurate assessment.**

Quality control

Fetal measurements should be accurate. Check your own performance regularly to make sure that your examinations are consistent:

1. Make any of the required measurements. Take the transducer off the patient. Repeat the measurement several times. Check the variation between the results.

2. Make the three standard measurements (crown–rump length, biparietal diameter and femur length). If possible, ask a colleague to repeat the examination on the same day on the same patient. Compare the results.

3. Compare your estimated delivery date with the actual date on which the baby is born. Do this for several babies.

4. Do the quality control tests routinely, e.g. on the first Monday of each month, or on some other easily remembered day (see also pp. 40–41).

Scanning a patient for another physician

If you scan patients for a referring doctor, you must inform him or her of the range of accuracy of any information you provide. It is very important to let the referring doctor know how much to trust the ultrasound results.

Requests for specific measurements should not be carried out if the results will provide misleading or inaccurate information. For example, a request to measure the biparietal diameter at 36 weeks to determine the exact gestational age is not acceptable, because the measurement has a large range of variation at that time and the result will be inaccurate. Choose whatever measurement is most appropriate for the period of the pregnancy, and give the doctor the information required after using the most accurate method.

> **There are limits to the accuracy of ultrasound. Use clinical, laboratory and serial measurements (at intervals of 2 weeks or more) when assessing fetal development.**

Normal pregnancy

Scanning a normal pregnancy must follow a strict routine, with identification of uterine and fetal anatomy.

The following routine is recommended:

1. Survey the maternal lower abdomen and pelvis.
2. Locate the fetus.
3. Assess the fetal head (including the skull and brain).
4. Assess the fetal spine.
5. Assess the fetal chest.
6. Assess the fetal abdomen and genitalia.
7. Assess the fetal limbs.

Normal pregnancy

The first ultrasound examination should include a survey scan of the whole of the lower maternal abdomen. The commonest finding is of corpus luteum cysts, which are usually less than 4 cm in diameter until the 12th week (Fig. 184a). Very large cysts may rupture, causing haemorrhage (Fig. 184b). There may also be torsion of the ovary.

The uterine adnexa and all the contents of the pelvis should be routinely surveyed for any abnormality, particularly scarring, a large ovarian cyst or large myoma (see pp. 210–211) which may interfere with pregnancy. If found, these should be measured and followed up (p. 235).

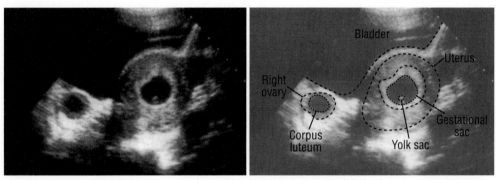

Fig. 184a. Typical appearance of a corpus luteum cyst in the right ovary, with an intrauterine (8 weeks) gestational sac.

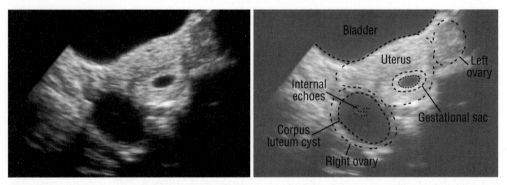

Fig. 184b. A large corpus luteum cyst (more than 4 cm) of the right ovary, with low-level internal echoes. Although most likely due to haemorrhage, these echoes have no clinical significance.

Ultrasound examination during pregnancy should include a systematic evaluation of fetal anatomy.

Apart from anencephaly, the fetal organs cannot be accurately measured before 17–18 weeks of gestation. After 30–35 weeks, evaluation becomes increasingly difficult.

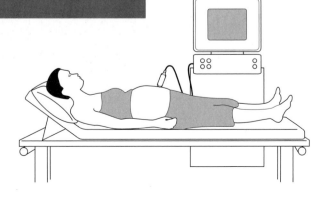

Examine the uterus to:

1. Locate the fetus or fetuses.
2. Locate the placenta.
3. Determine the orientation of the fetus.
4. Estimate the amount of amniotic fluid.

Fetal head

> ## The most important part of prenatal ultrasound is the assessment of the fetal head.

Ultrasound can demonstrate the fetal head by the eighth week of gestation, but intracranial anatomy becomes visible only after 12 weeks.

Technique

Scan the uterus to locate the fetus and the fetal head. Position the transducer at the side of the fetal head and do axial sections from the fetal vertex down to the base of the skull.

First locate the "midline echo", a linear echo that runs from the frontal to the occipital fold of the fetal head. It is due to the falx cerebri, the midline fissure between the two halves of the brain, and to the septum pellucidum. If the scan is just below the top of the head, the midline echo appears to be continuous and is due to the falx. Lower down there is an anechogenic rectangular area anteriorly in the midline which is the first gap in the continuous midline echo. This is the cavum septi pellucidi. Just behind and below this septum are two relatively anechogenic areas, the thalami. Between them are two closely parallel lines, the lateral walls of the third ventricle (these are seen only after the thirteenth week) (Fig. 185).

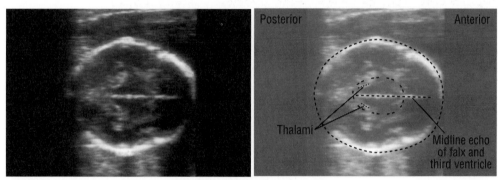

Fig. 185a. The normal midline echo of the falx cerebri.

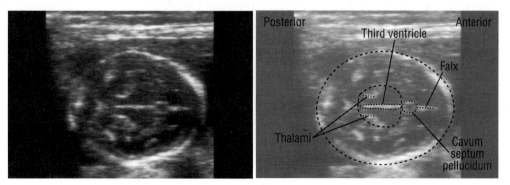

Fig. 185b. The cavum septi pellucidi at 21 weeks' gestation. The thalami are hypoechogenic.

At a slightly lower level, the middle of the lateral ventricle lines disappears, but the frontal and occipital horns are still visible (Fig. 186).

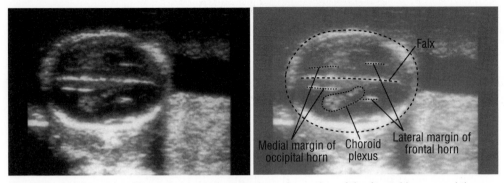

Fig. 186. Axial scan: at 20 weeks' gestation, the lateral margins of the frontal horns and the medial margins of the occipital horns are visible.

The choroid plexuses will be seen as echogenic structures filling the lateral ventricles. The frontal and occipital horns of the ventricles contain fluid, but no choroid plexus (Fig. 187).

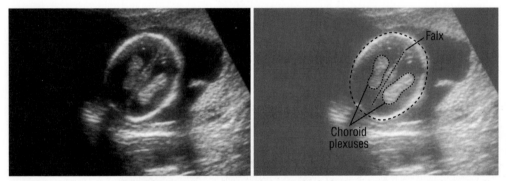

Fig. 187. Axial scan: the head of a normal fetus at 17 weeks' gestation showing the choroid plexuses filling the lateral ventricles.

Scan 1–3 cm lower (caudally) close to the upper part of the brain stem to locate a heart-shaped structure of low echogenicity with the apex pointing occipitally. Just in front will be the pulsations of the basilar artery and further forward again the pulsating circle of Willis should be seen.

Posterior to the brain stem is the cerebellum, which is not always visible. If the obliquity of the section is changed, the falx will still be visible (Fig. 188).

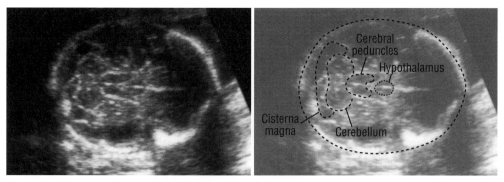

Fig. 188. The cerebellum, cisterna magna, cerebral peduncles, and hypothalamus.

Below this the next scan will show the base of the skull which appears x-shaped. The anterior branches of the cross are the sphenoid wings; the posterior branches are the petrous pyramids of the temporal bones.

The ventricles are measured above the level of the BPD. Look for the complete midline falx and then two straight lines that are close to the midline anteriorly and move further away posteriorly. These are cerebral veins and mark the lateral wall of the lateral ventricles (Fig. 189). Echogenic structures in the ventricles correspond to the choroid plexus.

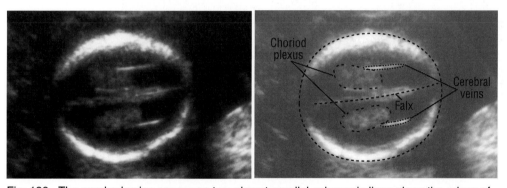

Fig. 189. The cerebral veins appear as two almost parallel echogenic lines along the edges of the lateral ventricles.

To assess the size of the ventricles, calculate the ratio of the width of the ventricle to the width of a hemisphere at the widest part of the skull. Measure the ventricle from the middle of the midline echo to the lateral wall of the ventricle (the cerebral vein). Measure the hemisphere from the midline to the inner table of the skull. The value of this ratio changes as the fetus grows, but is normal if less than 0.33. Higher values need to be compared with the normal range for the gestational age. Ventriculomegaly (usually hydrocephalus) requires further investigation and follow-up ultrasound. The infant should also be evaluated in the early neonatal period.

In the front of the skull it is easy to recognize the fetal orbits; the lenses of the eyes will appear as bright dots anteriorly (Fig. 190a). If the correct scan can be obtained, the fetal face can be seen in the axial (Fig. 190b) or coronal (Fig. 190c) planes. Movement of the mouth and tongue can be observed after 18 weeks.

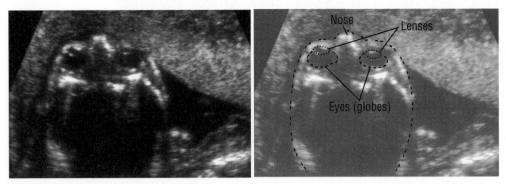

Fig. 190a. Axial scan showing the fetal orbits, the eyes and the lenses: the lenses are focally echogenic, but the globes are otherwise anechogenic.

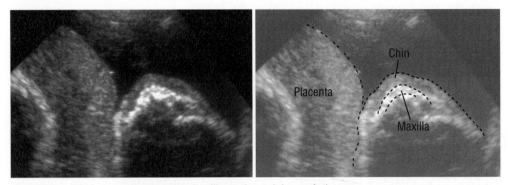

Fig. 190b. Axial scan showing the maxilla and overlying soft tissues.

If the position of the fetal head permits, make a sagittal scan anteriorly to visualize the frontal bone, maxilla, mandible and mouth (Fig. 190c).

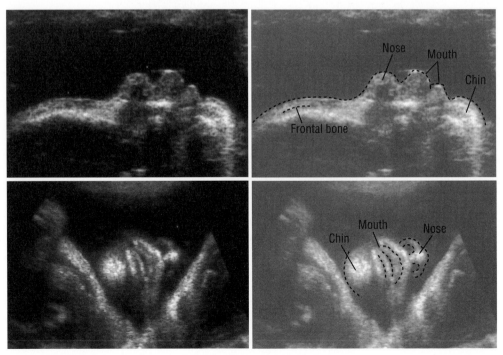

Fig. 190c. Sagittal (upper) and coronal (lower) scans: the lower part of the face is clearly seen.

Check that all the facial structures are symmetrical and appear normal, looking especially for cleft palate (this usually needs considerable experience) (Fig. 190d).

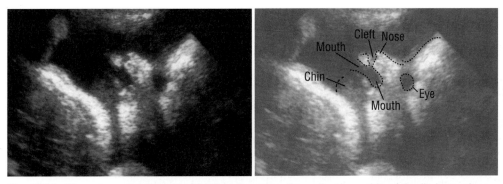

Fig. 190d. There is an asymmetrical cleft in the upper lip so that one side of the lip is much larger than the other. Cleft lips can also be symmetrical.

Scan the posterior portion of the skull and neck to rule out the rare meningocele or occipital encephalocele (pp. 263 and 264). Scanning from the midline to the side can also rule out cystic hygroma (Fig. 191). (Transverse scans of the posterior lower skull and neck are often easier.)

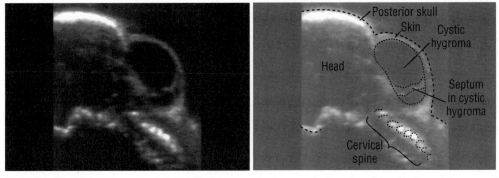

Fig. 191. Sagittal scan: a septate cystic hygroma in the cervical region. The skull, vertebrae and skin are normal.

Fetal spine

The fetal spine can usually be identified by the 12th week but can be clearly seen from the 15th week of gestation onwards. In the second trimester (12–24 weeks), the vertebral bodies have three separate ossification centres: the central one will form the anterior mass of the vertebra and the two posterior centres will form the laminae. These are seen as two strongly echogenic lines (Fig. 192a, b and c).

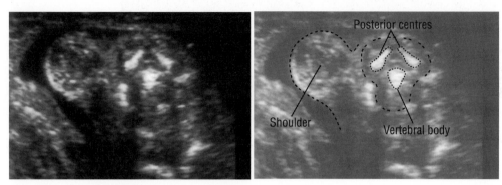

Fig. 192a. Transverse scan: the cervical spine.

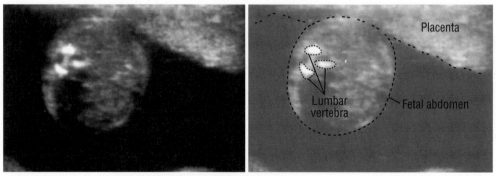

Fig. 192b. Transverse scan: the upper lumbar spine.

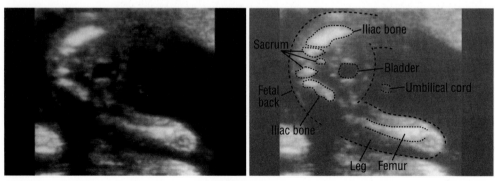

Fig. 192c. Transverse scan: the lumbosacral spine.

Although transverse scans will show the three ossification centres and intact skin over the spine, longitudinal scans are needed throughout the length of the spine to exclude defects or meningocele (Fig. 192d, e). Coronal scans may show clearly the relationship of the posterior ossification centres (Fig. 192f).

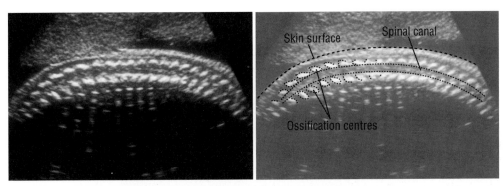

Fig. 192d. Longitudinal scan: the fetal spine at 22 weeks' gestation.

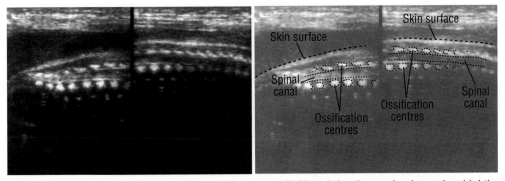

Fig. 192e. Longitudinal scans: the lumbosacral spine (left) and the thoracolumbar spine (right). The skin and the spinal canal can be seen.

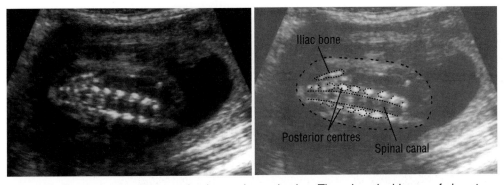

Fig. 192f. Coronal scan: the lower lumbar and sacral spine. There is a double row of almost parallel echoes arising from the posterior ossification centres.

Because of the curvature of the fetus, it is not easy to perform a longitudinal scan of the entire length of the fetal spine after 20 weeks.

Fetal chest

Transverse scans are the most useful for visualizing the fetal chest, but longitudinal scans can also be helpful. The exact level can be determined by recognizing the pulsation of the fetal heart.

Fetal heart

Fetal heart motion can be detected at 7–8 weeks' gestation but detailed anatomy can be seen only after 16–17 weeks. The fetal heart lies almost perpendicularly to the fetal trunk because it is pushed up by the relatively large liver. A transverse scan through the chest images the long axis of the heart and provides a view of all four cardiac chambers (Fig. 193). The right ventricle lies close to the anterior chest wall and the left ventricle close to the spine. The normal heart rate is 120–180 beats per minute, but transient slower rates may occur.

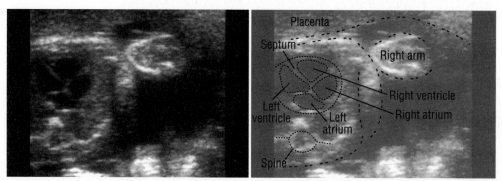

Fig. 193. The fetal heart at 31 weeks' gestation. The four cardiac chambers, the septa and the valves can be seen.

The cardiac chambers are about equal in size. The right ventricle is round with a thick wall, the left ventricle is more oval in shape. The atrioventricular valves should be visible and the intraventricular septum should be intact. The fluttering valve of the foramen ovale should be seen opening into the left atrium. (The heart is more clearly seen in the fetus than postnatally because the fetal lungs are not aerated and the heart can be scanned in different planes.)

Fetal lungs

The lungs can be seen as two homogeneous, moderately echogenic structures on either side of the heart (Fig. 194). They are not well developed until late in the third trimester and by 35–36 weeks their echogenicity should equal that of the liver and spleen. When this occurs it is probable that the lungs are reasonably mature, but maturity cannot be accurately assessed by ultrasound.

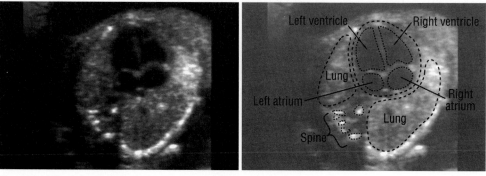

Fig. 194. The fetal heart and lungs. The lungs are echogenic and homogeneous. The heart is in early systole, so the atrioventricular valves are closed.

Fetal aorta and inferior vena cava

The fetal aorta can be seen on longitudinal scans (Fig. 195): look for the arch (with its major branches), the descending and abdominal aorta, and the bifurcation into the iliac vessels. The inferior vena cava can be visualized as a large vessel entering the right atrium just above the liver.

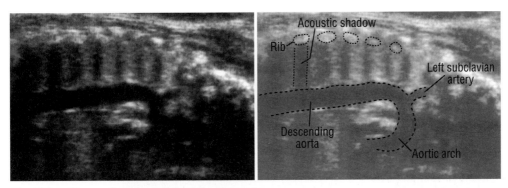

Fig. 195a. The aortic arch and the thoracic aorta.

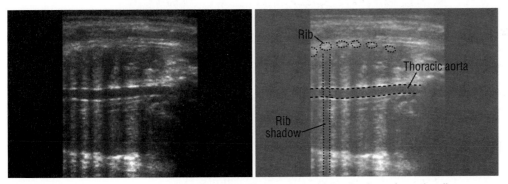

Fig. 195b. Coronal scan of the thoracic aorta. There are multiple shadows from the ribs.

Fetal diaphragm

On the longitudinal scans the diaphragm will show as a relatively hypoechogenic band between the lungs and the liver, moving during respiration. Both sides of the diaphragm should be identified. This may be difficult because it is very thin (Fig. 196).

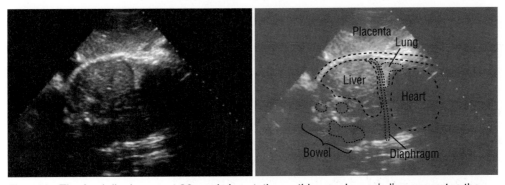

Fig. 196. The fetal diaphragm at 36 weeks' gestation: a thin anechogenic line separates the heart and lungs from the abdominal viscera. The lungs and liver have different echogenicities.

Fetal abdomen

Transverse scans through the fetal abdomen are the most useful for visualizing the abdominal organs.

Fetal liver

The liver fills the upper portion of the fetal abdomen. It is homogeneous in echogenicity and, until the last few weeks of gestation, is more echogenic than the lungs (Fig. 197).

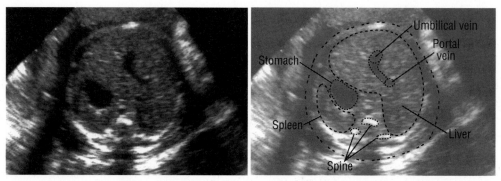

Fig. 197. Transverse scan showing the fetal liver, which is homogeneous, the left portal vein, spleen and the stomach.

Umbilical vein

The umbilical vein is seen as a small anechogenic tubular shadow and can be traced from its entrance at the midline of the abdomen upwards through the liver tissue and the portal sinus. The umbilical vein joins the ductus venosus at the sinus, but the sinus is not usually visualized as it is much smaller than the vein. If the position of the fetus permits, the insertion of the umbilical cord on the fetal abdomen should be located (Fig. 198).

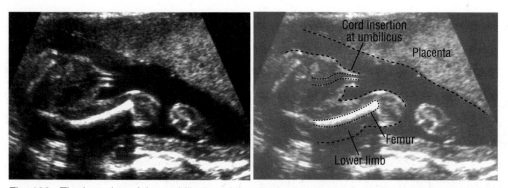

Fig. 198. The insertion of the umbilical cord into the fetal abdomen, with the vessels continuing on into the fetus.

> **Scan the fetal abdomen to visualize the site of cord insertion, and to confirm the continuity of the fetal abdominal wall.**

Fetal abdominal circumference

To obtain the circumference or the area of the fetal abdomen for the estimation of fetal weight, measure on a scan that shows the inner end of the umbilical vein at the portal sinus (see p. 239).

Fetal spleen

It is not always possible to image the spleen. When visible, it lies posteriorly to the stomach and is a semilunar, hypoechogenic structure (Fig. 197).

Fetal gallbladder

The fetal gallbladder cannot always be identified, but may be seen as a pear-shaped structure lying parallel to the umbilical vein on the right side of the abdomen (Fig. 199). Because they are close together in the same plane they can be mistaken for each other. However, the umbilical vein will pulsate and can be followed to other vessels. It should be localized first. The gallbladder lies to the right of the midline and ends at about a 40° angle to the umbilical vein. It cannot be traced from the surface into the liver.

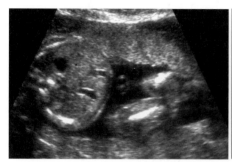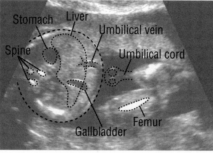

Fig. 199. The fetal abdomen: the gallbladder, lying next to the umbilical vein, is anechogenic. The stomach and liver can be seen.

Fetal stomach

The normal fetal stomach appears as a fluid-filled structure in the left upper quadrant of the abdomen (Fig. 200). It will vary in size and shape depending on the ingestion of amniotic fluid (Fig. 197, 199, 202): it is normally very active with peristaltic movement. If, in a fetus of 20 weeks or older, the stomach is not seen after 30 minutes' observation, it may be that the fluid level is low, the stomach absent or malpositioned (e.g. in a congenital diaphragmatic hernia), or the stomach and oesophagus are not connected (e.g. in tracheo-oesophageal fistula).

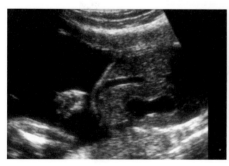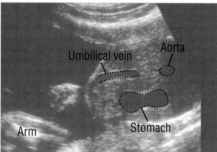

Fig. 200. Transverse scan of the fetal abdomen at the level of the umbilical vein, showing the stomach and part of the aorta.

Fetal intestine

Multiple fluid-filled loops of bowel can be seen in the second and third trimesters. The colon is usually seen just below the fetal stomach, and is predominantly anechogenic and tubular. Haustra may be identified. The colon is best seen in the last few weeks of pregnancy.

The small bowel is central. The colon is peripheral.

Fetal kidneys

The kidneys may be imaged from 12–14 weeks onwards, but will only be routinely seen clearly after 16 weeks. In transverse section they appear as hypoechogenic, circular structures on either side of the spine (Fig. 201). Within them can be seen the strongly echogenic renal pelvis; the capsule is also echogenic. The renal papillae are hypoechogenic and can appear large. Some dilatation of the renal pelvis (less than 5 mm) may sometimes be seen but is a normal finding. It is important to assess renal size by comparing the renal circumference with the abdominal circumference.

> **The normal ratio between the kidney and abdominal circumferences is 0.27–0.3.**

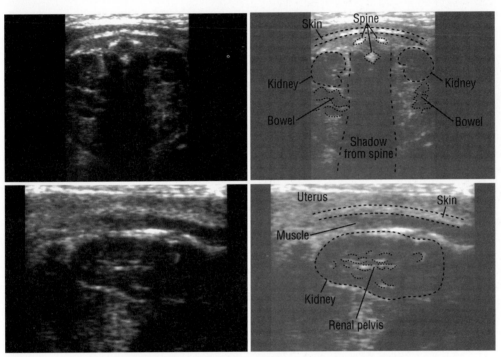

Fig. 201. The normal fetal kidney in transverse (upper) and longitudinal (lower) scans: the kidney tissue is hypoechogenic, but the renal capsule and pelvis are echogenic.

Fetal adrenal/suprarenal glands

The adrenals can be visualized only after the 30th gestational week, and will then be seen as relatively hypoechogenic structures above the upper poles of the kidneys. They are ovoid or triangular in shape and may be up to half the size of the normal kidney (this is much larger than in the neonate) (Fig. 202).

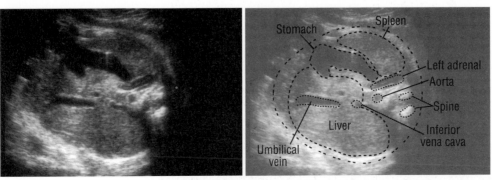

Fig. 202. Transverse scan: the fetal abdomen, showing the left adrenal gland and stomach.

Fetal urinary bladder

The bladder is a small ovoid cystic structure and can be recognized within the pelvis as early as 14–15 weeks. If not immediately seen, it may be identified on repeat scanning 10–30 minutes later. If the change in size can be assessed, it should be noted that normal urinary production at 22 weeks is 2 ml per hour, whereas at full term it is 26 ml per hour (Fig. 203).

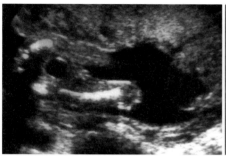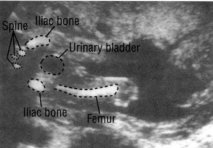

Fig. 203. The fetal urinary bladder shown as a cystic structure within the fetal pelvis.

Fetal genitalia

Male genitalia can be more easily recognized than female. The scrotum and penis may be seen as early as 18 weeks, but the female genitalia can only be reliably identified after 22 weeks. The testes are seen in the scrotum in the third trimester, unless there is a mild hydrocele (a normal variation) in which case they may be seen earlier (Fig. 204a).

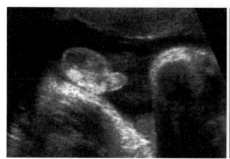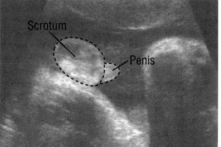

Fig. 204a. The male genitalia.

The labia majora and minora in the female become visible on the transverse scan of the perineal area from 23 weeks onwards (Fig. 204b).

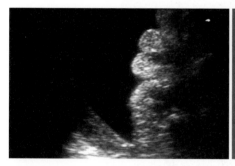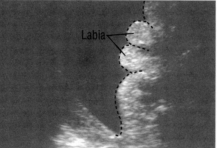

Fig. 204b. The female genitalia at 28 weeks' gestation. It is not always easy to recognize the labia.

Recognition of the fetal sex by ultrasound is of no importance unless there is a sex-linked congenital anomaly or a multiple gestation, when it is wise to determine zygosity and locate the placenta.

The patient should *not* be informed of the sex of the fetus until after 28 weeks, even though it may have been recognized earlier.

Fetal limbs

The fetal extremities can be seen from the 13th week of gestation. Each of the fetal limbs should be identified and the position, length and movement noted: this examination can take quite a long time.

The ends of the fetal limbs are the most easily recognized. The proximal bones can be clearly seen and the digits can be seen earlier than the carpus and tarsus, which ossify after birth. The fingers and toes become identifiable after 16 weeks. Evaluation of the feet and hands for anomalies is very difficult.

The long bones are dense compared with other structures. The femur is the most easily seen because of the limited movement of the thigh; the humerus is more difficult. The lower part of each limb (tibia and fibula, radius and ulna) is the least easily visualized (FIg. 205).

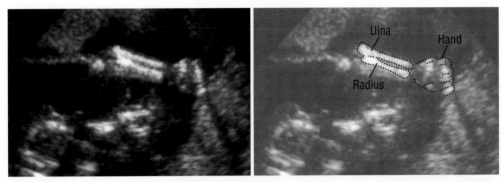

Fig. 205a. The normal fetal arm and hand. Fetal movement may make it difficult to see small details of the limbs.

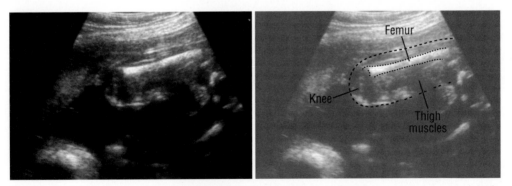

Fig. 205b. A full-length image of a fetal femur. The knee joint is flexed.

Fetal femur

The easiest way to find a femur is to scan longitudinally down the fetal spine to the sacrum: one of the femurs will then be recognized. The transducer should then be slowly angled until the entire length is imaged and can be measured (see pp. 38 and 240).

> **When measuring the length of a bone, it is important to be sure that the complete bone is seen: if the scan is not along the axis, the measurement will be shortened.**

The abnormal fetus

Fetal anomalies

Neurological anomalies

- Anencephaly
- Hydrocephaly
- Microcephaly
- Encephalocele

Spinal anomalies

- Myelomeningocele
- Spina bifida

Cystic hygroma

Cardiac anomalies

- Malposition
- Ventricular septal defect
- Hypoplasia

Gastrointestinal anomalies

- Duodenal atresia
- Jejunal atresia
- Cardiac atresia

Abdominal wall defects

- Omphalocele
- Gastroschisis
- Fetal ascites

Renal anomalies

- Hypoplasia
- Obstruction
- Cystic disease

Amniotic fluid

- Oligohydramnios
- Polyhydramnios

Fetal death

Neurological anomalies

1. **Anencephaly**—absence of the vault of the skull and brain—is the most common anomaly of the fetal central nervous system. It can be recognized at 12 weeks' gestation; there will be hydramnios and there may be other anomalies (Fig. 206). The α-fetoprotein is usually elevated in the amniotic fluid and maternal serum (see also pp. 270–271).

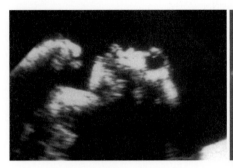
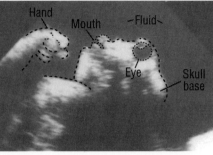

Fig. 206. Anencephaly: the face and the base of the skull are visible, but the rest of the head is missing. There is excess amniotic fluid (polyhydramnios).

2. **Hydrocephalus** can be recognized by the 18th week of gestation. There will be dilatation of the anterior and posterior horns of the lateral ventricles (Fig. 207a). For normal brain scans, see pp. 247–249.

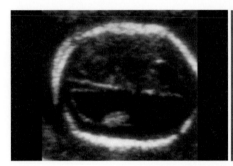
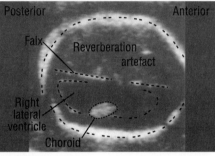

Fig. 207a. Hydrocephalus: the right lateral ventricle is dilated and the choroid plexus has dropped to the dependent side. Reverberation artefact obscures the left lateral ventricle.

Hydrocephalus due to the Arnold-Chiari malformation is associated with a lumbar myelomeningocele. The frontal bossing gives the head a characteristic shape which should always initiate a detailed evaluation of the fetal head and spine, particularly if the maternal serum α-fetoprotein is elevated.

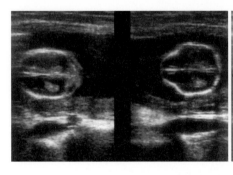
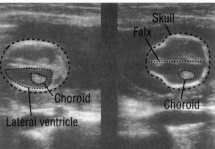

Fig. 207b. Hydrocephalus, due to Arnold-Chiari malformation. The scan on the left shows the hydrocephalus; on the right is the characteristic shape of the head associated with this malformation.

If the hydrocephalus is secondary to brain atrophy, the head is usually smaller than normal (Fig. 207c).

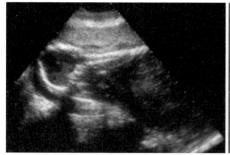 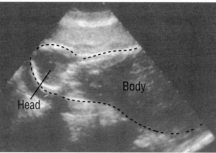

Fig. 207c. Microcephaly: the fetal head is much smaller than it should be for the size of the body.

3. **Microcephaly**. An abnormally small head can be diagnosed when the biparietal diameter is more than three standard deviations below the normal (see pp. 237–238). The biparietal diameter must be measured, but it is also essential to calculate the head:body ratio to exclude intrauterine growth retardation (see pp. 241–243). Isolated microcephaly, without other anomalies, is rare and the diagnosis can be difficult in borderline cases. Serial examinations and very careful interpretation are necessary. Except when the head is very small, do not diagnose microcephaly unless there are other anomalies.

Be *very* cautious with the ultrasound diagnosis of microcephaly. Serial examinations are essential.

4. **Encephalomeningocele**. This neural tube defect is characteristically seen as a circular sac protruding from the bony calvaria and containing fluid or brain tissue (Fig. 208). The occiput is the commonest site, but anterior encephaloceles are common in some ethnic groups. When asymmetrical, evidence of amniotic bands should be sought. The commonest source of error is the similar shadow caused by the fetal ear or by a limb alongside the head. Repeat scans in different planes and at different times may be necessary. Confusion may be caused by cystic hygroma, but the calvaria will be intact. Encephaloceles may be associated with infantile polycystic kidneys and polydactyly.

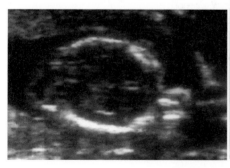 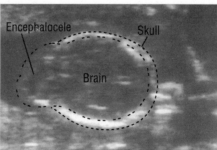

Fig. 208. An encephalocele (containing both neural tissue and cerebrospinal fluid) protrudes in the midline posteriorly.

Recognition of neurological anomalies can be extremely difficult. They should always be confirmed by repeat scans and preferably by another observer.

Spinal anomalies

Spinal anomalies are most common in the cervical and lumbar spine. The soft tissue overlying the spine should be examined for continuity, and the fetal spine for malformation. The fetal spine can be clearly seen from the 15th week of gestation onwards.

Myelomeningocele appears as a fluid-containing sac posteriorly, often with neural elements (Fig. 209 upper). An open myelomeningocele may have no sac, only disruption of the soft tissue over the defect: unraised defects are the most difficult to detect. A bony abnormality can usually be seen. Normally posterior ossification centres appear as two echogenic, near-parallel lines, but spina bifida will cause the lines to diverge. On normal transverse scans the posterior elements appear parallel; with spina bifida, the posterior elements are laterally displaced, not parallel, and pointing outwards (Fig. 209 lower). Longitudinal scans are particularly useful in detecting the protruding sac.

> **Not all degrees of spina bifida can be recognized by ultrasound.**

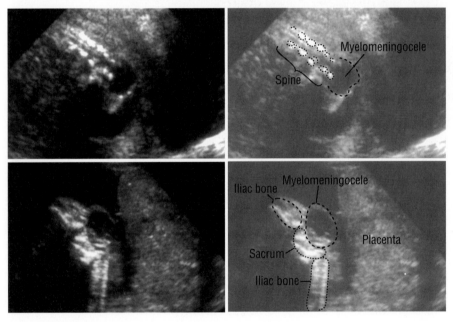

Fig. 209. Coronal (upper) and transverse (lower) scans of a myelomeningocele. There is a cystic mass protruding posteriorly from the lumbosacral spine. The neural elements cause internal echoes.

Cystic hygroma

Cystic hygroma is an abnormality of the lymphatic system, a cystic mass with septations, found in the neck posteriorly. It may extend laterally and anteriorly (Fig. 210), sometimes with a central septation or "spoke-wheel" aspect. Unlike encephalocele or cervical meningocele, the skull and spine are intact.

When cystic hygroma is associated with a generalized lymphatic anomaly and fluid collects in the chest or abdomen, survival is unlikely.

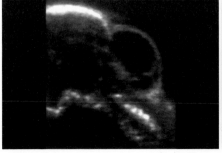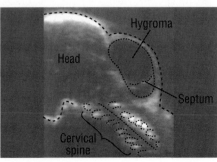

Fig. 210. A septate cystic hygroma in the cervical region. The skull, vertebrae and skin are normal.

Fetal cardiac anomalies

The detection of most cardiac anomalies requires sophisticated equipment and special training, including Doppler examinations. Malposition, hypoplasia of one side and ventricular septal defects may be seen, but if cardiac abnormalities are suspected, expert opinion should be obtained. If referral is not possible, the obstetrician or attending physician should be warned of the suspected abnormality and be present at the birth.

Fetal gastrointestinal anomalies

Congenital intestinal obstruction most commonly occurs either in the duodenum or in the jejunum and ileum.

1. **Duodenal atresia** is the commonest anomaly of the gastrointestinal tract. There will be two round cystic structures in the upper abdomen of the fetus. The "cyst" on the left is the dilated stomach, the one on the right is the duodenum. This is the "double-bubble" sign. Hydramnios is present in 50% of the cases associated with Down syndrome, and often there are also cardiac, renal and central nervous system anomalies (Fig. 211).

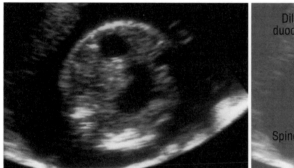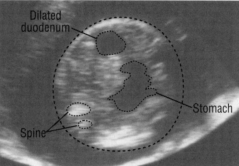

Fig. 211. Duodenal atresia, associated with hydramnios. Peristalsis could be seen in the stomach and in the dilated proximal duodenum.

2. **Jejunal-ilial atresia**. The diagnosis may be difficult. Multiple cystic structures will be seen in the upper fetal abdomen; these are dilated loops of bowel (Fig. 212). They are not usually seen until the second routine scan (in the third trimester). Hydramnios may be present when there is obstruction high in the gastrointestinal tract, but not when it is in the distal bowel. Associated anomalies are not as common as with duodenal atresia.

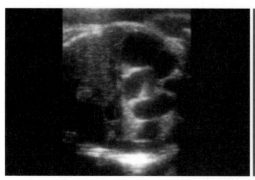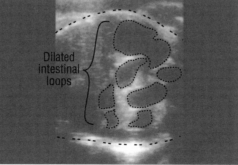

Fig. 212. Ilial atresia, causing marked dilatation of the small intestine.

If intestinal obstruction is suspected, repeat the scan in a few days to confirm the findings.

3. **Colonic obstruction or atresia**. This condition is rare and the diagnosis difficult to make with certainty with ultrasound.

Fetal abdominal wall defects

The commonest defect in the abdominal wall is in the midline (omphalocele); this is often associated with other congenital anomalies. Depending on the size of the defect, the hernia may contain part of the bowel, liver, stomach and spleen, covered by a membrane of amnion externally and parietal peritoneum internally. The umbilical vessels usually insert into the hernia sac and can be seen spreading within the sac wall (Fig. 213a).

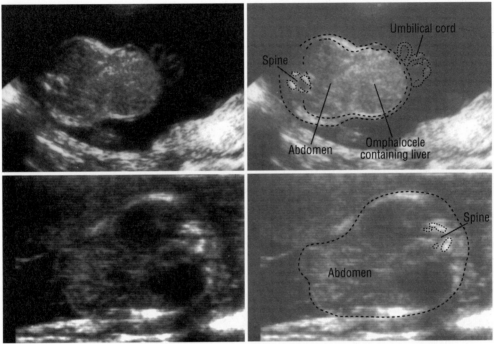

Fig. 213a. Omphalocele (upper) and pseudo-omphalocele (lower). Upper: the liver and bowel protrude through the defect where the umbilical cord is inserted into the abdominal wall. Lower: the prominent bulge is the result of compression of the fetal abdomen; it later disappeared. The antenatal diagnosis of an omphalocele must always be confirmed by scanning in different positions and at different times.

Other defects occur mainly in the right periumbilical region (gastroschisis), and are usually isolated. Only the bowel bulges through these periumbilical defects and there is no covering membrane. Ultrasound will show loops of bowel floating in the amniotic fluid outside the abdominal wall. The umbilical cord inserts normally (Fig. 213b).

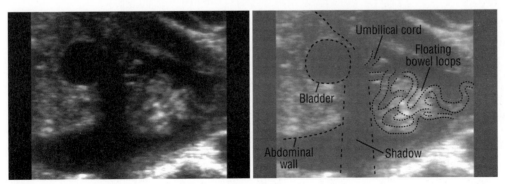

Fig. 213b. Gastroschisis: there is free-floating bowel, not covered by peritoneum, anterior to the abdominal wall. The umbilical cord insertion is normal.

Fetal ascites

Free fluid within the fetal abdomen can be recognized ultrasonically as an echo-free area surrounding the fetal viscera (Fig. 214). True ascites surrounds the falciform ligament and the umbilical vein, but pseudo-ascites is a hyopechogenic band surrounding the abdomen caused by abdominal musculature and fat.

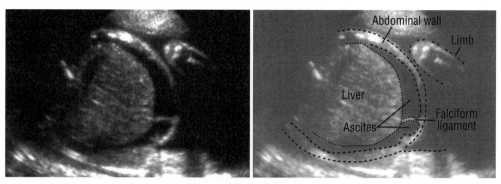

Fig. 214a. Fetal ascites, separating the liver from the abdominal wall. The skin is not thickened.

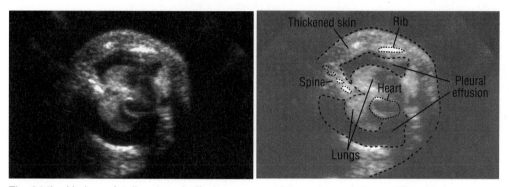

Fig. 214b. Hydrops fetalis: pleural effusions surround the echogenic lungs. The skin is thickened.

When ascites is suspected, the fetal anatomy should be carefully evaluated for associated anomalies. The major causes of ascites are renal obstruction and hydrops. Since ascitic fluid may be urine, the kidneys should be carefully scanned whenever there is ascites. Hydrops fetalis should not be diagnosed with certainty unless there is thickening of the skin (Fig. 214b, c) or more than one site of fluid collection (i.e. ascites with pleural or pericardial effusions). The common causes of hydrops are:

- Rhesus isoimmunization or other blood incompatibilities.
- Cardiac anomalies.
- Cardiac arrhythmias (typically tachyarrhythmias).
- Vascular or lymphatic obstruction (e.g. associated with cystic hygroma).

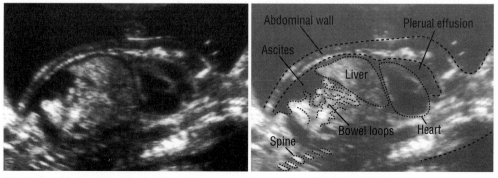

Fig. 214c. Hydrops fetalis: fetal ascites, separating the liver from the abdominal wall. The skin is thickened and there is also fluid in the chest.

Fetal urinary tract anomalies

Some renal anomalies are invariably fatal and, if recognized before 22 weeks of gestation, can be an indication for therapeutic abortion (where permissible). Recognition of the anomalies later in pregnancy can also influence management.

> **Even if the kidneys appear normal in echogenicity, size, shape and position, this does not exclude a urinary anomaly.**

1. **Renal agenesis (absent kidneys) syndrome.** There is no amniotic fluid and ultrasound is difficult. In the last few weeks of pregnancy, the kidneys may be thought to be present because the adrenal glands grow to a large size and become similar to the kidney in shape (Fig. 215). The bladder is usually small or absent. Scan at many different angles.

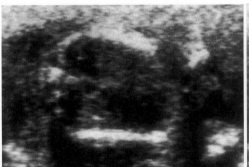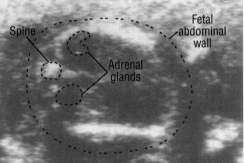

Fig. 215. Renal agenesis, with severe oligohydramnios. The large, hypoechogenic adrenal glands have filled the renal fossae.

2. **Hypoplastic (small) kidneys.** Renal measurements may show that the kidneys are small.

3. **Renal obstruction; hydronephrosis.** It is important to remember that transient dilatation of the renal pelvis can occur. Such dilatation is usually bilateral but can be unilateral, and may persist for some time (p. 258). Repeat the scan after two weeks. If the dilatation of the renal pelvis is physiological, either there will be no change or it may disappear.

    If the dilatation is pathological, it will usually worsen (Fig. 216a). Bilateral renal obstruction (hydronephrosis) is usually associated with a decrease in the amount of amniotic fluid (oligohydramnios) and has a poor outcome. Unilateral obstruction is not associated with a decrease in amniotic fluid because the other kidney provides adequate renal function.

    In some cases there will actually be increased fluid (hydramnios). On ultrasound, an increased cystic echo-free space will be seen in the centre of the kidneys (or kidney) with smaller cysts budding outwards. The presence of these small cysts (less than 1 cm) on the cortical surface of hydronephrotic kidneys is a reliable but infrequent sign of dysplasia (Fig. 216a, b). Increased echogenicity and diminished cortical thickness are less reliable signs of inadequate function.

    If the obstruction is at the level of the ureteropelvic junction, close to the kidney, the renal pelvis tends to be rounded, and dilated ureters will not be seen. When there is obstruction at the bladder outlet (usually due to urethral valves in males), the bladder, as well as both ureters and both renal pelves, may be dilated (Fig. 216c, d). Sometimes the distended posterior urethra may be seen as an outpouching from the urethra.

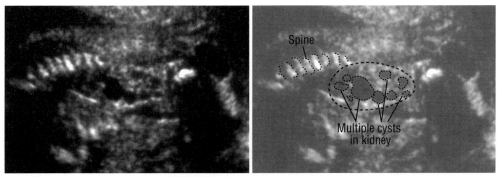

Fig. 216a. Multicystic kidney with oligohydramnios: the cortical cysts were less than 1 cm in diameter. There were other fetal anomalies.

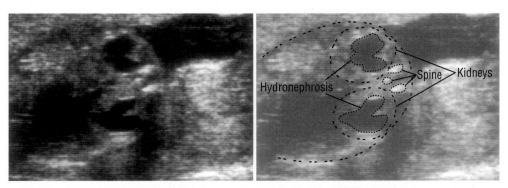

Fig. 216b. Transverse scan showing bilateral hydronephrosis. The renal cortex is normal.

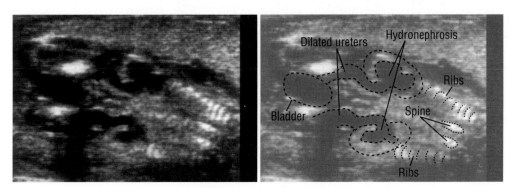

Fig. 216c. Coronal scan: bilateral hydroureter and hydronephrosis, caused by bladder outlet obstruction. The bladder did not empty even after one hour.

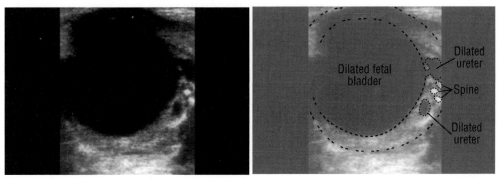

Fig. 216d. Marked dilatation of the fetal bladder as a result of urethral obstruction. The kidneys and ureters were dilated.

4. **Multicystic kidney.** Scans will show several cysts of different sizes, usually scattered but rarely in one part of one kidney. The condition is fatal if in both kidneys. Renal tissue may be visible between the cysts, there is no clearly defined renal cortex, and the tissue will be more echogenic than normal renal parenchyma (Fig. 217).

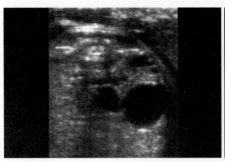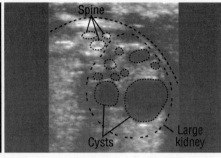

Fig. 217. A multicystic kidney: the other kidney was completely normal.

5. **Autosomal recessive renal polycystic disease** is not usually recognized until the third trimester. A family history is usually known and there will be oligohydramnios because of poor urinary secretion. Both kidneys may be so large that they resemble the liver except for their shape. The individual cysts are too small to be seen by ultrasound, but there are so many interfaces that the kidney becomes strongly echogenic (Fig. 218).

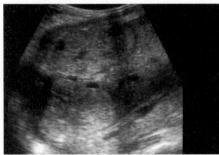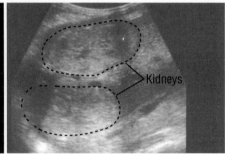

Fig. 218. Bilateral polycystic kidneys at 34 weeks' gestation. The kidneys are hyperechogenic but the individual cysts are too small to be imaged by ultrasound scanning.

Amniotic fluid

1. **Increased amniotic fluid (hydramnios, polyhydramnios).** Increased amniotic fluid may be seen in a number of conditions that affect the fetus. The most common causes are:

   - Gastrointestinal obstruction (high jejunal or more proximal) (Fig. 219).
   - Central nervous system anomalies and neural tube defects.
   - Hydrops fetalis.
   - Some abdominal wall defects.
   - Small-chested skeletal dysplasias (dwarfisms), which are usually fatal.
   - Twins.
   - Maternal diabetes.

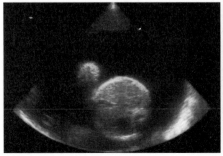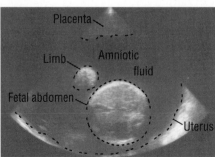

Fig. 219. Polyhydramnios at 36 weeks' gestation. The fetus had oesophageal atresia.

2. **Decreased amniotic fluid (oligohydramnios).** Fetal urinary secretion is mainly or entirely responsible for amniotic fluid production from 18–20 weeks onwards. If there is bilateral renal obstruction, dysplasia or non-functioning kidneys, the amniotic fluid may be significantly diminished or absent (Fig. 220). This will lead to pulmonary hypoplasia.

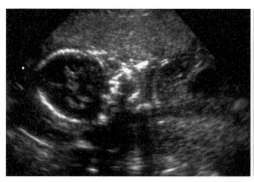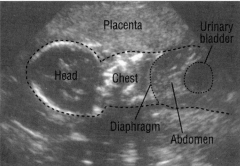

Fig. 220. Oligohydramnios. The fetal head and body are close to the uterine wall and placenta. The urinary bladder is dilated as a result of outlet obstruction.

The etiology may be:

- Rupture of the membranes with a leak of fluid.
- Bilateral renal or urinary outlet anomaly (either urethral or affecting both kidneys or ureters).
- Intrauterine growth retardation.
- Postmaturity.
- Fetal death.

- **The majority of masses within the fetal abdomen are of renal origin.**

- **Multicystic kidneys may be unilateral or bilateral and have non-communicating cysts.**

- **Autosomal recessive (infantile) polycystic disease appears as solid echogenic kidneys: single cysts will not be recognized.**

- **Oligohydramnios is a poor prognostic feature when there is a fetal renal anomaly because it is associated with pulmonary insufficiency.**

Fetal death

The diagnosis of fetal death is made when there is no cardiac motion. There may be transient bradycardia or pauses in heart motion in normal fetuses, and observation should last for several minutes. Other signs of death are oligohydramnios and collapse of the skull with overriding of the skull bones (Spalding's sign) (Fig. 221).

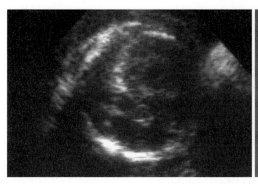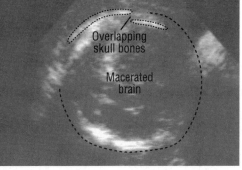

Fig. 221. Fetal death: the bones of the skull overlap, there is oligohydramnios and no cardiac movement could be seen on real-time scanning.

Placenta

> **Examination of the placenta is an *essential* part of any obstetric ultrasound examination.**

The placenta is essential to fetal well-being, growth and development; it can be demonstrated reliably and accurately by ultrasound. The exact position can be determined relative to the fetus and the internal os of the uterine cervix. The structure of the placenta and the utero-placental junction can be assessed.

> **Uterine contractions can mimic the placenta or a mass in the uterine wall (see p. 273).**

Scanning technique

The patient should have a full, but not over-distended, bladder so that the lower section of the uterus and the vagina can be clearly seen. Ask her to drink 3 or 4 large glasses of water before the examination.

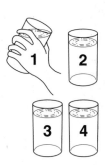

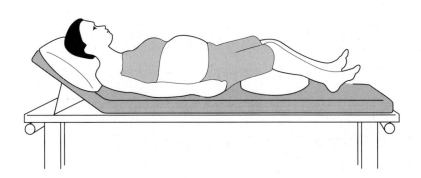

Multiple longitudinal and transverse scans will be necessary to demonstrate the placenta completely. Oblique scans may also be needed.

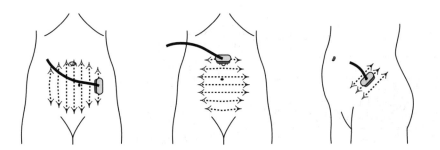

Normal placenta

At 16 weeks' gestation the placenta occupies half of the inner surface of the uterus. At 36–40 weeks' gestation, the placenta occupies 1/4 to 1/3 of the inner surface area of the uterus (see pp. 274–276).

Uterine contractions can mimic the placenta (Fig. 222a) or a mass in the uterine wall (Fig. 222b). Repeat the scan after 5 minutes, but remember that contractions can last a surprisingly long time. If in doubt, wait longer (p. 235).

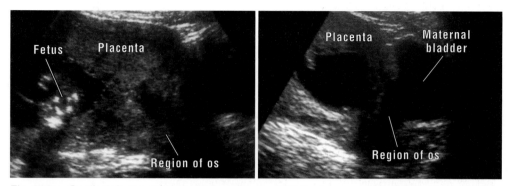

Fig. 222a. On the left, the placenta appears to cover all the lower portion of the uterus. A later scan (right) shows that the contraction had relaxed and the edge of the placenta is well away from the internal os.

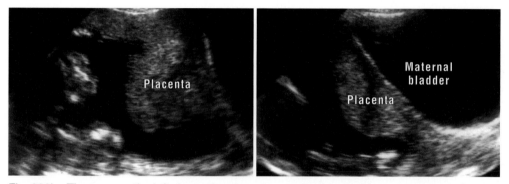

Fig. 222b. The scan on the left shows the placenta apparently raised by a mass; several minutes later (right) the contraction has resolved and the mass has disappeared. Unlike a myoma, a contraction is homogeneous, hypoechogenic and does not extend outside the uterus.

> **Accurate and prompt localization of the placenta is very important in patients with vaginal bleeding or with signs of an unstable fetus, particularly in the later stages of pregnancy.**

> **An overdistended bladder can sometimes produce a false impression of placenta praevia (p. 274). Ask the patient to partially empty her bladder and then repeat the examination.**

Placental location

From 14 weeks onwards it is easy to locate the placenta (Fig. 223). Oblique scans may be necessary for a posteriorly situated placenta.

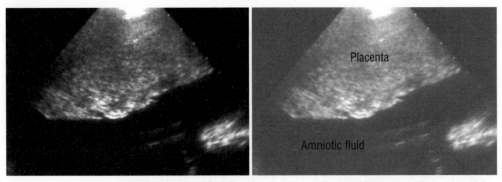

Fig. 223. At 26 weeks' gestation the normal placenta is smooth and almost homogeneous.

The placental position is described in relation to the walls of the uterus and the cervical os. Its position may therefore be right, midline or left. If the placenta is free of the os, its position from front to back may be described as anterior, anterofundal, fundal, posterofundal or posterior.

Placenta praevia

Identification of the internal cervical os is critical to the diagnosis of placenta praevia. The cervical canal may be seen as an echogenic line surrounded by two hypoechogenic or anechogenic lines, or it may be entirely hypoechogenic (Fig. 224). The cervix and lower uterine segment will appear different whether the bladder is full or empty. With a full bladder the cervix appears elongated; edge shadows from the fetal head, bladder or pubic bone may obscure some detail. When the bladder is less full, the cervix changes orientation to become more vertical and perpendicular to the sound beam. Although the cervix is more difficult to find when the bladder is empty, it is less distorted, and the relationship of the placenta to the internal cervical os can be more accurately determined.

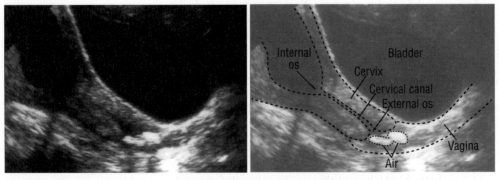

Fig. 224. The normal uterine segment and cervix: the cervical canal is hypoechogenic, surrounded by two hyperechogenic lines. There is air in the vagina, causing bright echoes, following a pelvic examination.

> **A diagnosis of placenta praevia, made when the bladder is full, should be confirmed by rescanning when the bladder has been partially emptied.**

Placental position

1. If the placenta covers the os completely, there is *central* placenta praevia (Fig. 225a).

2. If the edge of the placenta covers the os, this is *marginal* placenta praevia (but the os is still entirely covered by the placenta) (Fig. 225b).

3. If the lower edge of the placenta is close to the os, this is a *low-lying* placenta (Fig. 225c). This diagnosis can rarely be made with any accuracy, since it is difficult to determine if only a part of the os is covered by the placenta.

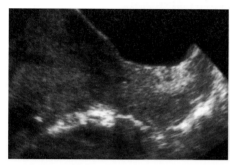
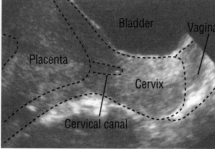

Fig. 225a. Central placenta praevia: the os is completely covered. The maternal urinary bladder is full.

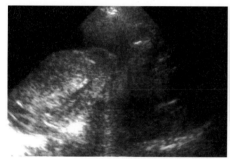
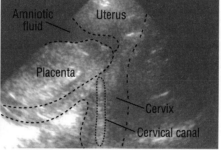

Fig. 225b. Marginal placenta praevia: the internal os is covered by the edge of the placenta. The maternal urinary bladder is empty and the cervix lies almost vertically.

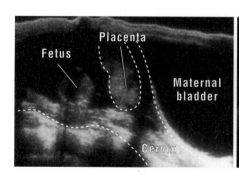
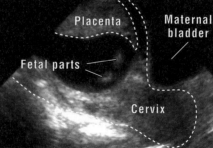

Fig. 225c. Pseudo placenta praevia: on the left, the placenta appears to cover the lower segment of the uterus. After partial emptying of the bladder (right), it can be seen that the placental edge is not near to the internal os.

The location of the placenta may appear to change during pregnancy if it is evaluated only when the bladder is full. Re-examination with a partially empty bladder is necessary.

Placenta praevia may be identified during the early months of pregnancy and not seen at term. However, a central placenta praevia recognized at any time, or a placenta praevia identified at or after 30 weeks, is unlikely to change significantly. Provided there has been no bleeding in the second trimester, a second routine scan can be delayed to 36 weeks to confirm the diagnosis. If there is any doubt, the examination should be repeated before 38 weeks or before labour.

Normal placental pattern

The placenta may be homogeneous or may have indentations or echogenic foci along the basal plate (Fig. 226a). Echogenic septa extending across the width of the placenta may be seen in the later stages of pregnancy.

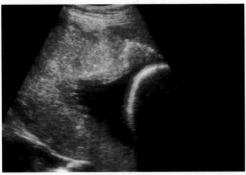
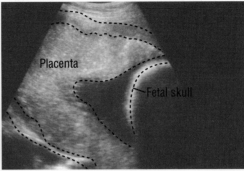

Fig. 226a. A normal placenta.

Anechogenic areas immediately beneath the chorionic plate or within the placenta frequently result from thrombosis and subsequent accumulation of fibrin (Fig. 226b). When not extensive they can be considered normal.

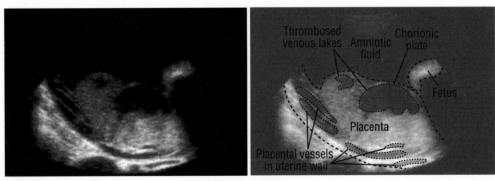

Fig. 226b. Large uterine vessels should not be mistaken for abruptio placentae. In this patient, there is also thrombosis in the venous lakes below the chorionic plate.

Intraplacental anechogenic areas may be caused by moving blood seen in dilated vascular spaces. If they involve only a small part of the placenta, they are of no clinical concern.

Under the basal plate of the placenta, retroplacental hypoechogenic channels may be seen along the wall of the uterus as a result of venous drainage (Fig. 226c). This should not be mistaken for a retroplacental haematoma (p. 278).

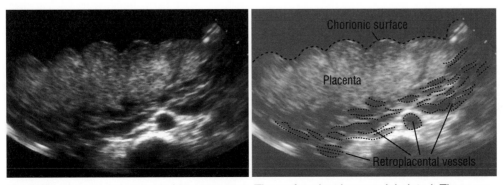

Fig. 226c. A normal placenta in late pregnancy. The surface has become lobulated. There are retroplacental veins, which must not be mistaken for a haematoma.

Abnormal placental patterns

Hydatidiform mole can be readily diagnosed by its typical "snow-storm" pattern (Fig. 227) (see p. 234). It is important to note that the fetus may still be present and only part of the placenta may be affected.

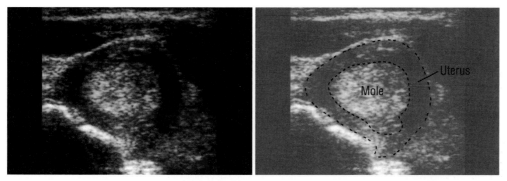

Fig. 227. Transverse scan: the uterus is filled with speckled echoes, the "snow-storm" appearance typical of hydatidiform mole.

Enlarged (thick) placenta

Measurement of the placental thickness is too inaccurate to influence clinical decision-making. Any assessment can only be subjective (Fig. 228).

1. Enlargement of the placenta occurs in maternal–fetal rhesus incompatibility or hydrops.
2. Diffuse enlargement of the placenta may be seen in mild or moderate maternal diabetes.
3. The placenta is usually large if there is an infection involving the pregnancy.
4. The placenta may be large in abruptio placentae (see p. 278).

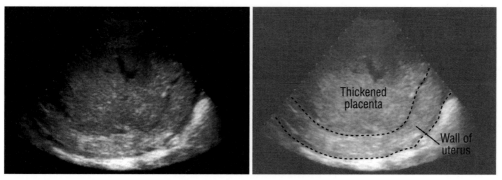

Fig. 228. A thick placenta (hydrops) due to maternal–fetal rhesus incompatibility.

Small placenta

1. The placenta is usually small and thin if the mother has insulin-dependent diabetes.
2. The placenta may be small when there is maternal pre-eclampsia or intrauterine growth retardation.

Abruptio placentae

Ultrasound is not a sensitive method for diagnosing abruptio placentae. Characteristically, there is a hypoechogenic or anechogenic area beneath or lifting the edge of the placenta (Fig. 229a). Blood may sometimes be seen separating the membranes (see also p. 276).

The haematoma may be echogenic and is sometimes so echogenic that it blends with the normal placenta (Fig. 229b). Apparent thickening of the placenta may be the only sign of a haemorrhage, or the placenta may appear normal.

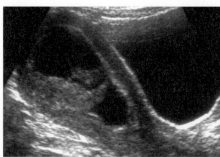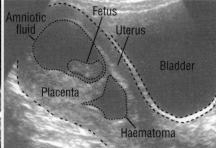

Fig. 229a. A retroplacental haematoma lifting the margins of the placenta. The haematoma eventually resolved.

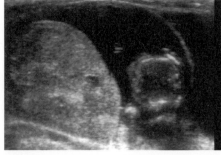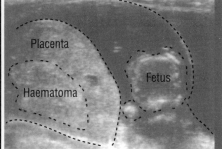

Fig. 229b. An echogenic retroplacental haematoma which blends with the placenta. It is only because the placenta appears so thick that haemorrhage can be suspected.

> **Ultrasound is not very accurate in the diagnosis of abruptio placentae. The clinical diagnosis remains very important.**

Incompetent cervix

Any separation (widening) of the os, indicating incompetence, should be identified. If there is fluid inside the cervix, the internal os may be identified by small knuckles of tissue projecting towards one another at right angles to the orientation of the cervix. The amniotic membrane may prolapse (Fig. 230). The bladder should be emptied to take pressure off the os, and a scan should determine if fetal parts or the umbilical cord have also prolapsed. The patient's hips should be raised and she should immediately be evaluated clinically.

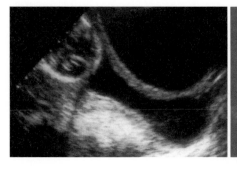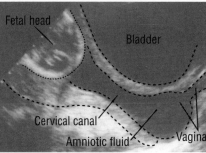

Fig. 230. An incompetent cervix: the amniotic membrane and fluid have prolapsed into the vagina through the open os.

The umbilical cord and vessels

The umbilical cord can be recognized in the first trimester, extending from the chorion frondosum to the fetal pole (Fig. 231a). Longitudinal and transverse scans will demonstrate one umbilical vein and two umbilical arteries. If there are only two vessels, it is always an artery that is missing: there will then be a high risk of perinatal mortality, and anomalies will occur in approximately 20% of fetuses (Fig. 231b).

There is also a high risk of intrauterine growth retardation when there is only one artery. Growth should be assessed at every scan (p. 242).

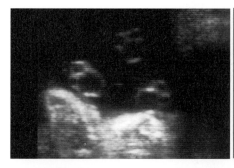 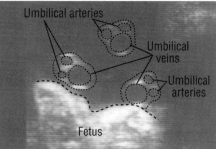

Fig. 231a. Transverse scan: the two umbilical arteries and one vein found in a normal umbilical cord.

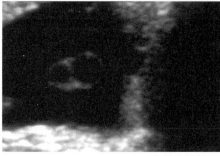 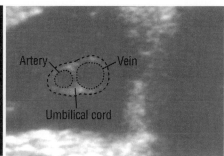

Fig. 231b. Transverse scan of an umbilical cord with only one artery and vein.

Multiple pregnancy

It is important to recognize each fetus and the position and number of the placentas in cases of multiple gestation. A separating membrane should be sought, usually most easily seen in the first or second trimester. If the fetuses are of different sex, there is dizygosity. The size of each fetus should be monitored to exclude a growth disturbance affecting only one. The amount of amniotic fluid in each sac should also be assessed (Fig. 232) (see also p. 231).

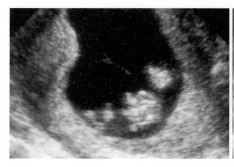 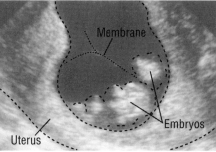

Fig. 232a. A first-trimester twin pregnancy, divided by a thin, but well defined membrane.

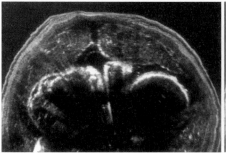 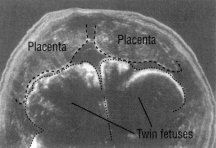

Fig. 232b. A twin pregnancy with two placentas, separated by a membrane which is only partially visible.

Summary: scanning during pregnancy

> **Many physicians believe there is no reason for any routine scans at any stage in a clinically normal pregnancy, and scan only when an abnormality is suspected on clinical examination. Other physicians believe that two routine scans are important for good antenatal care (p. 225).**

18–22 weeks' gestation

A scan at this stage will answer these questions:

1. Is it a single or multiple pregnancy?
2. Does the estimated age agree with the clinical gestational age?
3. Is the growth of the fetus normal for the gestational age?
4. Is the fetal anatomy normal?
5. Is fetal activity normal?
6. Is the uterus normal?
7. Is the amount of amniotic fluid normal?
8. What is the position of the placenta?

32–36 weeks' gestation

A scan at this stage will answer these questions:

1. Is the rate of growth normal for the period of gestation?
2. Is the fetus normal? Are there any developmental anomalies?
3. What is the position of the fetus (this may change before labour commences)?
4. What is the position of the placenta?
5. Is the amount of amniotic fluid normal?
6. Are there any complications, e.g. myomas, ovarian tumours, that might obstruct delivery?

Late in pregnancy

If the patient has not had a previous ultrasound scan and is in the last few weeks of pregnancy, a scan will answer these questions:

1. Is it a single or multiple pregnancy?
2. Does the fetal maturity match the clinical expectation?
3. What is the position of the fetus?
4. What is the position of the placenta? In particular, placenta praevia must be excluded.
5. Is the amount of amniotic fluid normal?
6. Are there any developmental anomalies?
7. Are there any complications, e.g. myomas, ovarian tumours, that might obstruct delivery?

Ultrasound before and after external cephalic version

An ultrasound examination is often necessary immediately before carrying out version from breech to vertex presentation to make sure that the fetus has not already changed position.

Following the version, ultrasound is useful to confirm that the fetal lie has become normal.

Ultrasound in early pregnancy (before 18 weeks)

If ultrasound scanning is considered necessary, it is preferable to wait until 18–22 weeks of gestation because this will provide the most useful information. However, there can be indications for ultrasound earlier during pregnancy, such as:

1. Vaginal bleeding.
2. Patient does not know the date of her last menstrual period or there is other reason for suspecting a discrepancy in dates.
3. There is no evidence of fetal life when expected.
4. There is a history of miscarriage, difficult labour or other obstetric or genetic problems.
5. An intrauterine device is known to be in place.
6. There is a reason for terminating pregnancy.
7. The patient is unduly anxious about the pregnancy.

Ultrasound at mid-pregnancy (28–32 weeks)

It is preferable to wait until 32–36 weeks for any necessary ultrasound examination, but there may be clinical indications for ultrasound earlier than this, such as:

1. Clinical problems with the position or size of the fetal head.
2. Clinical examination suggests an abnormality.
3. An earlier ultrasound was not entirely normal or satisfactory.
4. The placenta was not accurately localized or was close to the os during an earlier ultrasound examination.
5. The uterus is too large for the estimated gestational age.
6. There is leakage of amniotic fluid.
7. There is pain or bleeding.
8. The mother's clinical condition is unsatisfactory.

Indications and timing for additional ultrasound examinations

> **Ultrasound is unlikely to provide the explanation for mild or moderate abdominal pain unless there is evidence of pre-eclampsia.**

The following may be indications for additional ultrasound examinations:

1. Intrauterine growth retardation: repeat ultrasound after 2 weeks.
2. Low-lying placenta: repeat at 38–39 weeks and again if necessary before labour.
3. Abnormal presentation of the fetus: repeat at 36 weeks.
4. Discrepancy between the uterine size and gestational age: repeat at 36 weeks or earlier if the discrepancy is significant.
5. Known or strongly suspected fetal abnormality: repeat at 38–39 weeks.
6. Unexpected bleeding.
7. Lack of fetal movement or other evidence of fetal death: repeat ultrasound immediately and if there is any doubt, follow with further ultrasound in one week.

Ultrasound during labour

The indications for using ultrasound during labour are:

1. The position of the fetus is unstable.
2. The fetal heart cannot be detected clinically.
3. There is a discrepancy in the size of the pregnancy and the size of the fetus.
4. There is unusual bleeding.
5. Labour is delayed or is not following a normal clinical course.

Ultrasound in the postpartum period

There is no indication for a routine ultrasound examination following parturition, but there are some clinical findings that may suggest that ultrasound will provide further useful information.

In the immediate postpartum period:

1. Severe bleeding.
2. Retained placenta or torn placenta.
3. Undelivered twin or other fetus.

Six weeks postpartum:

1. Continued bleeding.
2. Persistent pain.
3. Failure of the uterus to return to normal size.
4. Continuous vaginal discharge.
5. Palpable mass in the pelvis.

CHAPTER 18

Neonates

> **Experience is needed to peform and interpret correctly all neonatal ultrasound examinations.**

Indications

Suspected anomalies of the:

1. Abdomen.
2. Head.
3. Hips.

For suspected pyloric stenosis, see p. 148.

Preparation for abdominal scans

1. **Preparation of the patient**. Clinical condition permitting, infants should be given *nothing* by mouth for 3 hours preceding the examination.

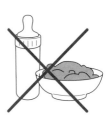

2. **Position of the patient**. The infant should be supine (on the back) on a soft, comfortable pillow. The arms should be lifted upwards so that the abdomen is extended.

   Cover the abdomen with coupling agent.

3. **Choice of transducer**. Use a 7.5 MHz transducer if available. However, satisfactory information can often be obtained with a 5 MHz transducer. Small sector transducers are preferable as they are more convenient for examining the small body of a neonate.

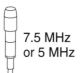

7.5 MHz
or 5 MHz

4. **Setting the correct gain**. Start by placing the transducer centrally at the top of the abdomen (the xiphoid angle). Angle the beam towards the right side of the patient to image the liver. Adjust the gain setting so that the image has normal homogeneity and texture. It should be possible to recognize the strongly reflecting lines of the diaphragm next to the posterior part of the liver and the portal and hepatic veins should be visible as tubular structures with echo-free lumens. The borders of the portal veins will have bright echoes, but the hepatic veins will not.

Scanning technique: abdomen

Both transverse and longitudinal scans are required. As in the adult, the aorta, inferior vena cava and portal veins should be identified (see p. 50).

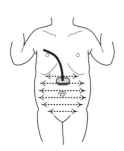
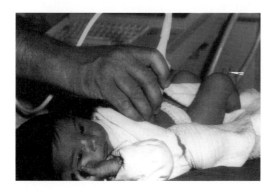
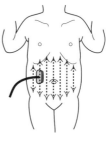

Neonatal abdomen

Indications

1. Abdominal mass.
2. Fever of unknown origin.
3. Haemolytic diseases.
4. Infections such as toxoplasmosis and listeriosis.

Liver

To see the whole liver as well as the liver parenchyma, the hepatic vein and the portal vein, multiple scans in different projections are required (Fig. 233).

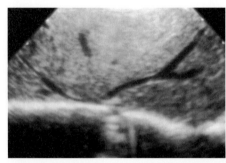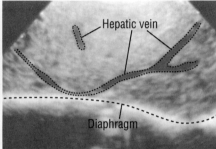

Fig. 233a. Transverse scan: normal hepatic veins.

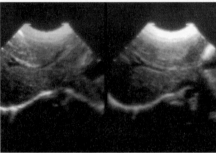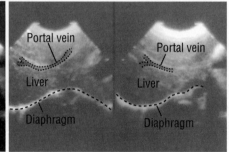

Fig. 233b. Transverse scan: normal portal veins.

Gallbladder (jaundice)

It is not always possible to distinguish between biliary atresia and neonatal hepatitis by ultrasound. Other causes of obstructive jaundice, such as a choledochal cyst, gallstones or inspissated bile, can be recognized. The normal neonatal gallbladder is 2–4 cm in length. It is usually absent or small in extrahepatic biliary atresia, but may be normal.

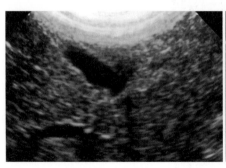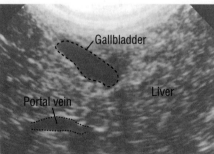

Fig. 234. Longitudinal scan: normal gallbladder in a neonate.

Blood vessels

It is important to demonstrate the major abdominal blood vessels and their main branches (Fig. 235).

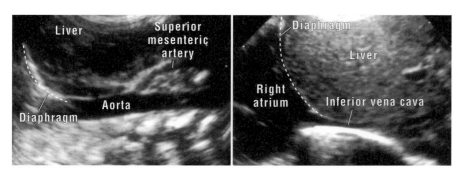

Fig. 235. Longitudinal scans. Left: the aorta and superior mesenteric artery. Right: the inferior vena cava and right atrium.

Kidneys

When scanning to exclude neonatal urinary disease, it is important to remember that, until the age of 6 months, neonatal kidneys differ acoustically from adult kidneys.

- The difference between the renal cortex and medulla is less marked in the infant.
- The renal pyramids are relatively hypoechogenic and may resemble cysts.
- The renal cortex is less echogenic than the liver parenchyma.

As the child grows older, the difference between the cortex and the medulla increases (Fig. 236).

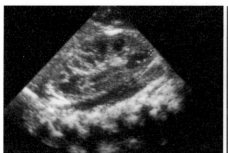
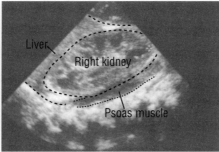

Fig. 236a. Longitudinal scan: a kidney just after birth.

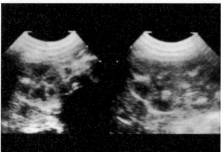
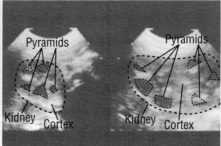

Fig. 236b. Transverse and longitudinal scans of an infant's kidney.

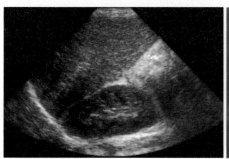
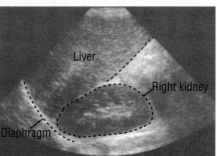

Fig. 236c. A kidney at the age of 6 years.

Intracranial sonography

> ## Intracranial sonography is not an easy examination.

Indications for neonatal cranial ultrasound:

1. Hydrocephalus (a large head).
2. Intracranial bleeding.
3. Hypoxaemic damage.
4. Meningocele and other congenital anomalies.
5. Convulsions.
6. A small head (microcephaly).
7. Bulging fontanelles (raised intracranial pressure).
8. Trauma.
9. Intrauterine infection.
10. After meningitis, to exclude aqueduct stenosis or other sequelae.

Scanning technique

Use a 7.5 MHz transducer if available; otherwise, use a 5 MHz transducer.

1st choice:
7.5 MHz

2nd choice:
5 MHz

Sagittal scan: centre the transducer over the anterior fontanelle with the scanning plane aligned with the long axis of the head. Angle the transducer first to the right, to see the right ventricle, and then to the left to see the left ventricle.

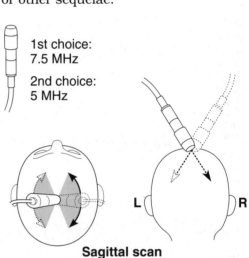

Sagittal scan

Coronal scan: rotate the transducer 90° so that the scan plane is aligned transversally, and angle the beam forward and then backward.

Posterior coronal scanning

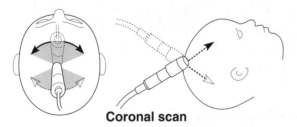

Coronal scan

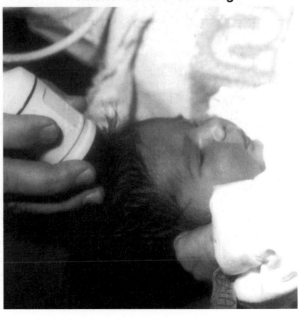

Axial scan: centre the transducer just above the ear and angle the beam up towards the vault and down towards the base of the skull. Repeat on the other side.

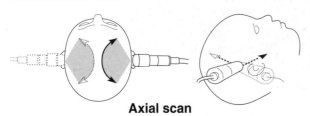

Axial scan

Normal midline anatomy

In 80% of neonates, the fluid-filled cavum septi pellucidi will be seen as a midline structure. Below the cavum will be the triangular fluid-filled third ventricle, and surrounding these structures will be normal brain tissue of varying echogenicity (Fig. 237).

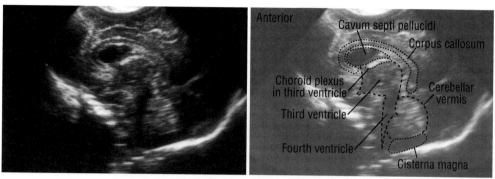

Fig. 237a. Midline sagittal scan: normal but premature neonatal brain.

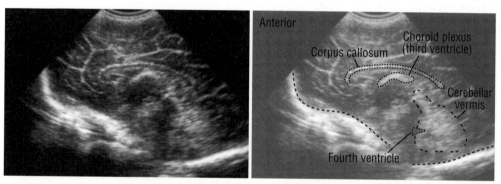

Fig. 237b. Midline sagittal scan: normal full-term neonatal brain.

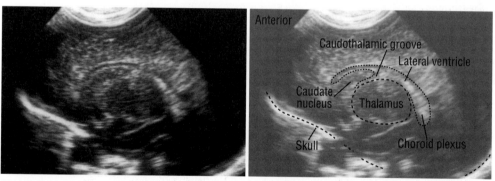

Fig. 237c. Angled left sagittal scan: normal lateral ventricle in a neonatal brain.

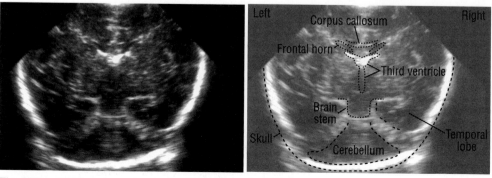

Fig. 237d. Midline coronal scan: the frontal horns of the lateral ventricles and the third ventricle of a neonatal brain.

Sagittal section

Angled sagittal sections on each side of the brain will show the lateral ventricles shaped like an inverted "U". It is important to visualize the solid thalamus and the caudate nucleus below the ventricles because this is the region of the brain in which haemorrhage is most frequent (Fig. 238).

By angling the transducer, the entire ventricular system can be examined.

The echogenic choroid plexus will be seen mainly within the atria and the temporal horns.

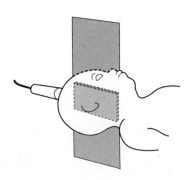

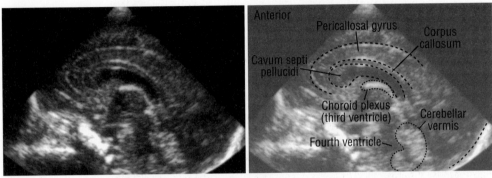

Fig. 238a. Midline sagittal scan: normal neonatal brain.

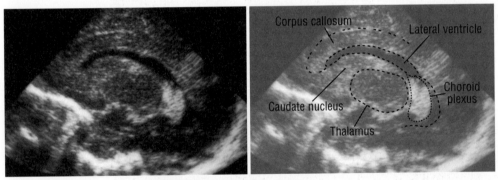

Fig. 238b. Sagittal scan angled 20° left: a normal neonatal brain.

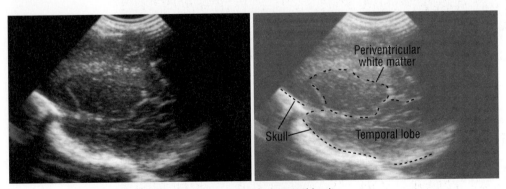

Fig. 238c. Sagittal scan angled 30° left: a normal neonatal brain.

Coronal section

Multiple scans should be performed at different angles, depending on the individual patient, to image the whole ventricular system and the adjacent brain (see diagram, p. 288). Use the most suitable angle for the particular part of the brain to be examined (Fig. 239).

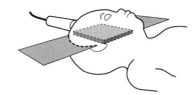

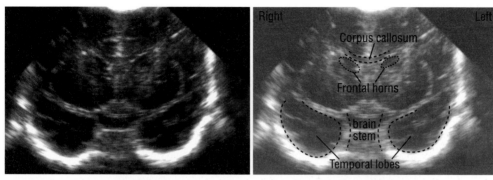

Fig. 239a. Coronal scan angled 10° anteriorly: a normal neonatal brain.

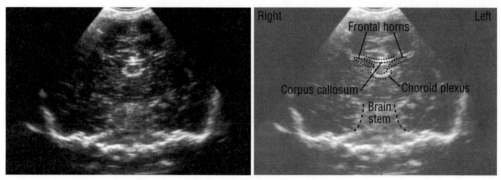

Fig. 239b. Midline coronal scan: a normal neonatal brain.

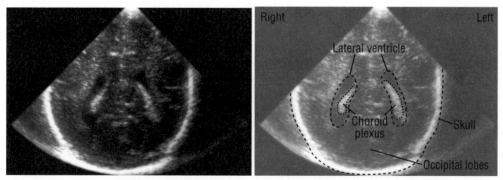

Fig. 239c. Coronal scan angled 20° posteriorly: a normal neonatal brain.

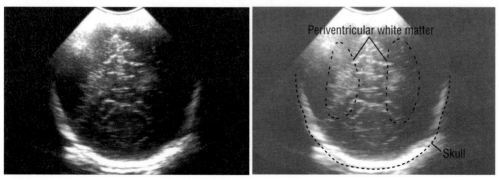

Fig. 239d. Coronal scan angled 30° posteriorly: a normal neonatal brain.

Axial section

The first, most inferior, section will demonstrate the heart-shaped pedicles and show arterial pulsation in the circle of Willis.

The next section above this will show the thalamus and the central echo of the falx cerebri (Fig. 240a, b).

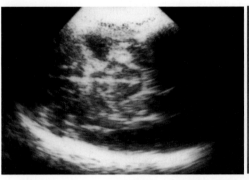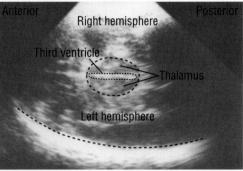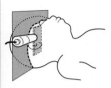

Fig. 240a. Axial scan from the right side: a normal neonatal brain.

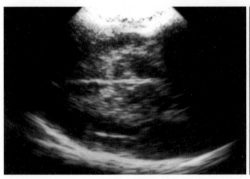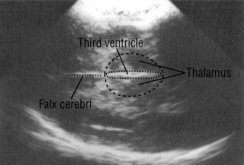

Fig. 240b. Axial scan from the right side: the thalamus, falx cerebri and third ventricle.

The top (superior) section will show the walls of the lateral ventricles. The ventricle and the corresponding hemisphere can then be measured (Fig. 240c).

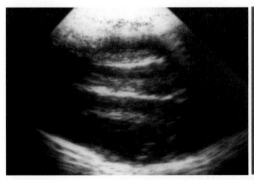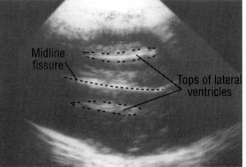

Fig. 240c. Axial scan from the right side: the lateral ventricles.

The ratio of the ventricle diameter to the hemispheric diameter should be less than 1:3. If it is greater, hydrocephalus must be considered.

$$\frac{\text{Ventricular diameter}}{\text{Hemispheric diameter}} \leq \frac{1}{3}$$

Ventricular dilatation

It is easy to recognize ventricular dilatation and asymmetry with ultrasound. If in doubt, re-examination after an interval is essential. One of the common causes of dilatation is congenital aqueduct stenosis (Fig. 241a, b).

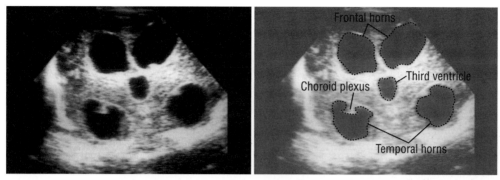

Fig. 241a. Coronal scan: dilated frontal and temporal horns of the lateral ventricles and dilated third ventricle.

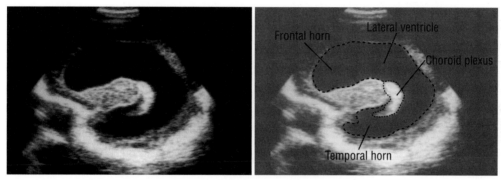

Fig. 241b. Sagittal scan angled 20° to the left: marked dilatation of the left ventricle.

Agenesis of the corpus callosum is another congenital cause of hydrocephalus. This causes marked lateral displacement of the lateral ventricles and upward movement of the third ventricle (Fig. 241c).

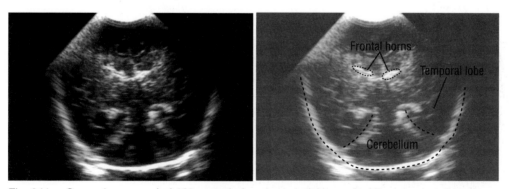

Fig. 241c. Coronal scan angled 10° posteriorly: agenesis (absence) of the corpus callosum.

Intracranial bleeding

1. **Subependymal bleeding** appears as one or more hyperechogenic areas just below the lateral ventricle, best seen in a transverse plane adjacent to the frontal horn. Confirm this with a sagittal scan: the haemorrhage may be bilateral. This is a grade I haemorrhage (Fig. 242).

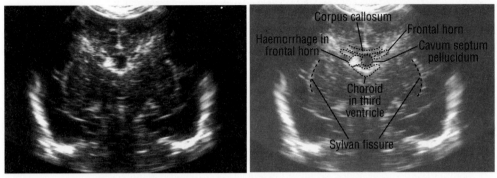

Fig. 242a. Coronal scan angled 10° anteriorly: grade I subependymal haemorrhage on the right side.

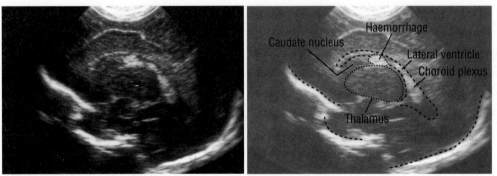

Fig. 242b. Sagittal scan angled 20° to the right: the same grade I haemorrhage as above.

2. **Intraventricular bleeding into normal size ventricles**. Additional echoes from the normally echo-free ventricles (as well as from the hyperechogenic choroid plexus) indicate thrombus (clot) in the ventricles. If there is no ventricular dilatation, this is a grade II haemorrhage (Fig. 242c).

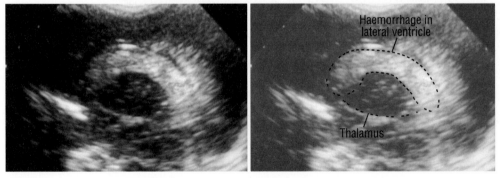

Fig. 242c. Sagittal scan angled 20° to the right: grade II haemorrhage into a normal-sized right ventricle.

3. **Intraventricular bleeding into dilated ventricles**. When there is intraventricular haemorrhage with ventricular dilatation, this is a grade III haemorrhage (Fig. 242d).

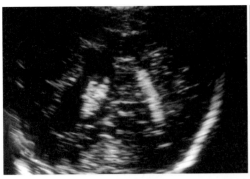
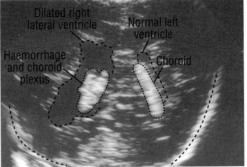

Fig. 242d. Coronal scan angled 20° posteriorly: grade III haemorrhage on the right side. The left side is normal.

4. **Intraventricular bleeding accompanied by bleeding into the brain substance** appears as areas of increased echogenicity within the brain. This is a grade IV haemorrhage, the most severe form (Fig. 242e).

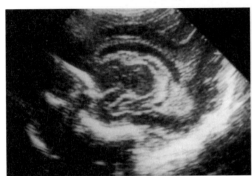
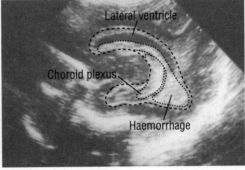

Fig. 242e. Sagittal scan angled 20° to the right: grade IV haemorrhage.

5. **Sequelae of bleeding**. In grades I and II, the blood is usually reabsorbed during the first week of life, but more severe bleeding (grades III and IV) can cause posthaemorrhagic hydrocephalus as well as loss of brain tissue (porencephalic cysts). Developmental retardation with abnormal neurological findings may result (Fig. 243).

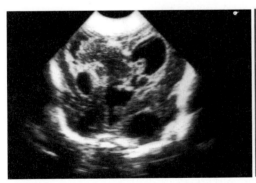
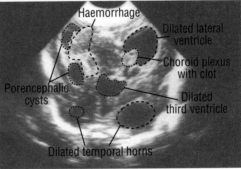

Fig. 243. Coronal midline scan: right-sided porencephalic cysts and hydrocephalus, the sequelae of a grade IV haemorrhage.

Neonatal cerebral abnormalities

- Necrosis of brain tissue results in a poorly delineated region of hypoechogenicity, usually lateral to the lateral ventricles (periventricular leukomalacia).

- Cerebral oedema can result in obliteration of the ventricle and of the cranial sulci. The brain is generally more echogenic than normal.

- Cerebral infections cause changes in echogenicity, including punctate hyperechogenic regions due to calcification.

Hips

Considerable skill and experience are needed to use ultrasound to diagnose dislocation of the hips in the neonate. With practice, it is possible to demonstrate the lower part of the iliac bone and the acetabulum, particularly the roof of the hip joint and the rim of the fossa. The exact position of the femoral head within the joint can be determined and any discrepancy in the shape or size of the hip joint can be imaged (Fig. 244).

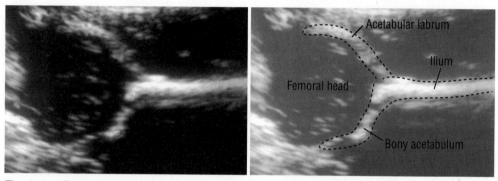

Fig. 244a. Coronal scan: normal newborn hip. The midplane line of the iliac bone normally bisects the femoral head.

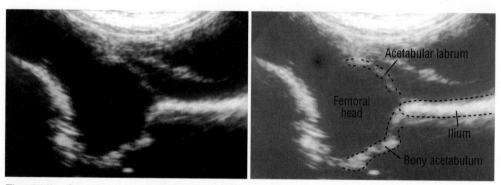

Fig. 244b. Coronal scan: newborn hip, shallow acetabulum. The bony acetabulum is not as deep as normal.

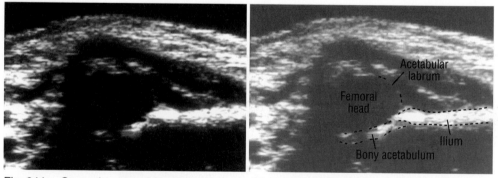

Fig. 244c. Coronal scan: subluxed newborn hip. The bony acetabulum is shallow and covers less than 50% of the femoral head.

When there is doubtful or very mild sonographic laxity in the hip of a newborn infant, repeat the scan at the age of 4–6 weeks. Many hips will have become normal by then.

CHAPTER 19

Neck

Indications

1. A palpable mass in the neck.

2. Abnormalities in the carotid arteries (a bruit or symptoms of carotid insufficiency). Doppler ultrasound is needed for a complete assessment.

> **Ultrasound is *not* a reliable way to exclude a parathyroid tumour.**

Preparation

1. **Preparation of the patient**. There is no specific preparation.

2. **Position of the patient**. The patient should be lying on his or her back (supine) with the neck extended over a pillow under the shoulders. The pillow should be about 10 cm thick.

   Apply coupling agent liberally to the neck.

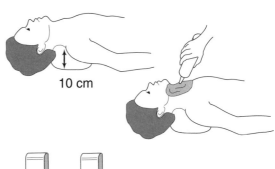

3. **Choice of transducer.** Use a 7.5 MHz linear transducer, if available; if not, use a 5 MHz linear or convex transducer.

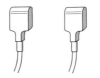

5 MHz   7.5 MHz

4. **Setting the correct gain**. Vary the gain to obtain the best image of the part being scanned.

Scanning technique

Scans should be done in both longitudinal and transverse planes, with oblique projections if necessary.

During the examination, it may be necessary to rotate the head from right to left, particularly for vascular studies.

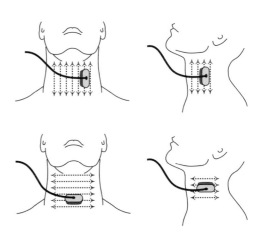

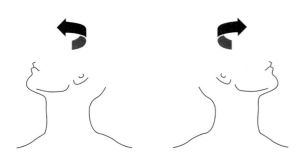

Normal anatomy

Ultrasound can demonstrate the following normal structures in the neck:

- Carotid arteries.
- Jugular veins.
- Thyroid gland.
- Trachea.
- Surrounding muscles.

It is important that all of these structures are located when scanning the neck.

1. **Vessels**. The vascular bundle (the carotid artery and the jugular vein) is behind and between the sternocleidomastoid muscle and lateral to the thyroid gland. These vessels are very accessible for ultrasonography.

   The carotid artery, bifurcating into the internal and external branches, will be seen as a tubular structure with hyperechogenic walls and an echo-free centre: the walls are smooth and difficult to compress with the transducer. The jugular vein is lateral to the carotid artery and the walls are more easily compressed (Fig. 246). The veins vary in diameter during the different phases of respiration and the Valsalva manoeuvre.

2. **Thyroid**. The thyroid consists of two lobes, one on either side of the trachea joined in the midline by an isthmus. The thyroid gland and the isthmus have the same homogeneous echo texture, and the lobes should be equal in size. On transverse scans, the section is usually triangular; on longitudinal scans, it is oval. The outline should be smooth and regular.

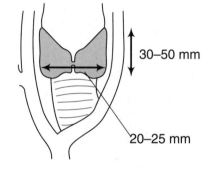

30–50 mm

20–25 mm

   The thyroid gland is normally 15–20 mm thick, 20–25 mm in width, and 30–50 mm in length (Fig. 247).

3. **Muscles**. The sternocleidomastoid muscle is the only muscle of particular importance in paediatric patients. The muscles are band-like structures which are less echogenic than the thyroid (Fig. 245). On transverse scans, the outline is well defined but varies from circular to ovoid in section.

4. **Lymph nodes**. Normal lymph nodes can sometimes be seen as hypoechogenic structures less than 1 cm in diameter.

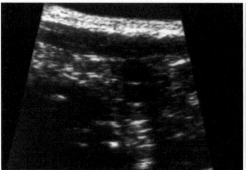
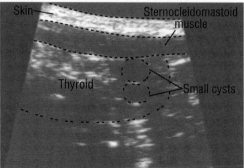

Skin — Sternocleidomastoid muscle

Thyroid — Small cysts

Fig. 245. Longitudinal scan: the thyroid gland and the sternocleidomastoid muscle. There are two small cystic masses in the thyroid.

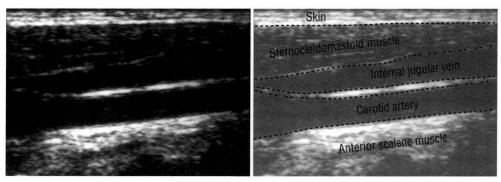

Fig. 246a. Longitudinal scan: the common carotid artery and the internal jugular vein.

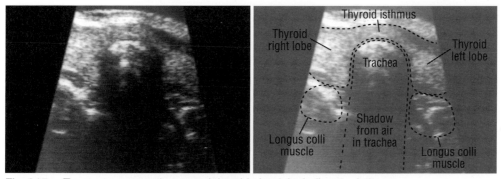

Fig. 246b. Transverse scan: the common carotid artery, jugular vein, thyroid gland and sternocleidomastoid muscle.

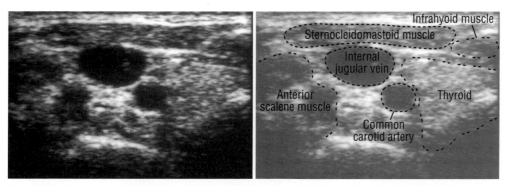

Fig. 247a. Transverse scan: the normal thyroid gland, including the isthmus.

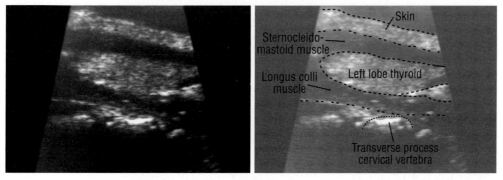

Fig. 247b. Longitudinal scan: normal thyroid gland.

Abnormal thyroid

Thyroid abnormalities may be local or diffuse, single or multiple.

Focal masses

1. **Solid.** About 70% of focal lesions are thyroid nodules and over 90% of these will be adenomas, which are very seldom malignant. The ultrasound appearance of an adenoma is variable and it may be impossible to differentiate between a benign thyroid adenoma and a malignant tumour: the ultrasound characteristics are similar, and size is not important. Both benign and malignant tumours can be hypo- or hyperechogenic; both may contain cystic components. However, if the mass is well circumscribed, with a surrounding thin, hypoechogenic halo, there is a 95% probability that it is a benign adenoma (Fig. 248a, b). When there is central necrosis, the possibility of malignancy should be considered (Fig. 248c).

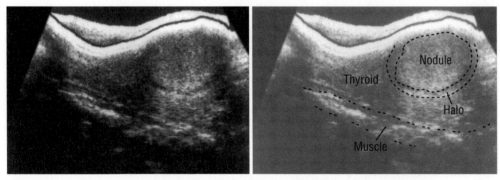

Fig. 248a. Longitudinal scan: an isodense nodule in the thyroid, surrounded by a hypoechogenic halo.

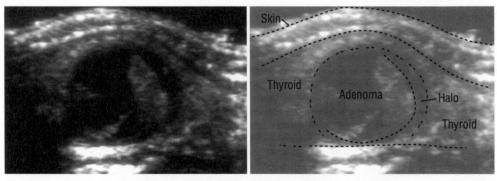

Fig. 248b. Longitudinal scan: a benign thyroid adenoma with cystic changes.

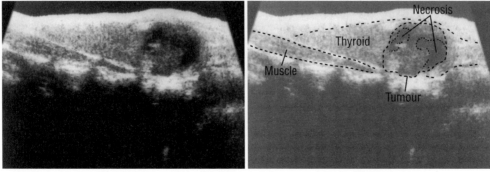

Fig. 248c. Longitudinal scan: carcinoma of the thyroid with central necrosis.

2. **Cystic**. True cysts of the thyroid are rare. Characteristically, they are well circumscribed, with smooth walls, and are echo-free, unless there has been haemorrhage into the cyst (Fig. 249).

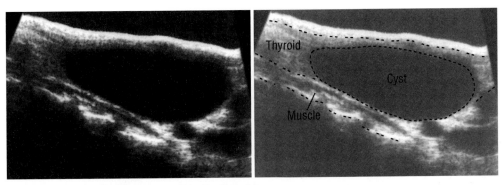

Fig. 249. Longitudinal scan: a cyst in the thyroid.

3. **Haemorrhage or an abscess** may occur in the thyroid, appearing as a cystic or complex pattern with ill-defined edges (Fig. 250).

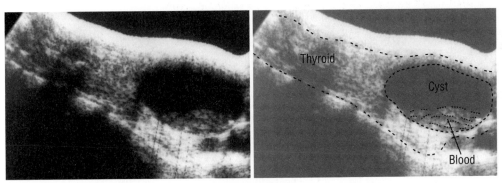

Fig. 250. Longitudinal scan: a thyroid cyst partially filled with blood.

4. **Calcification.** Ultrasound shows hyperechogenic areas with distal acoustic shadowing. Thyroid calcification is commonly seen in adenomas, but may occur in malignant tumours. The calcification can be isolated or in clusters, in groups or in chains. It is important to remember that the size of the thyroid nodule and the presence or absence of calcification are *not* evidence for or against malignancy (nor will radiological examination provide a better differential diagnosis) (Fig. 251).

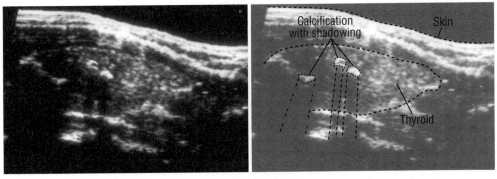

Fig. 251. Longitudinal scan: calcification in the thyroid gland.

A large thyroid gland with internal calcification *may or may not be malignant.* Neither ultrasound nor radiography can predict whether the mass is benign or malignant.

Diffuse thyroid lesions

Homogeneous enlargement

The thyroid may be enlarged, sometimes extending retrosternally. Enlargement may affect only part of a lobe, a whole lobe, the isthmus or both lobes. Enlargement is usually hyperplastic and is ultrasonically homogeneous. It may be due to endemic goitre, lack of iodine, puberty, hyperthyroidism or hyperplasia following partial thyroidectomy (Fig. 252a). A small, homogeneous, hypoechogenic thyroid may indicate acute thyroiditis.

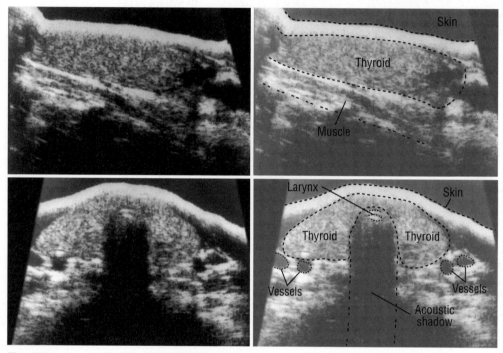

Fig. 252a. Longitudinal (upper) and transverse (lower) scans of homogeneous thyroid hyperplasia. The gland is hyperechogenic because of iodine deficiency.

Heterogeneous enlargement

If the ultrasound density of the thyroid is heterogeneous, there are usually multiple nodules (a multinodular goitre); the nodules may be solid or complex on ultrasound. (Fig. 252b, c). In autoimmune thyroiditis, the thyroid becomes heterogeneous and may resemble a multinodular goitre.

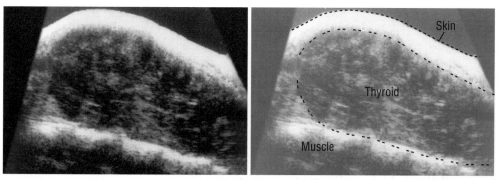

Fig. 252b. Heterogeneous hyperplasia of the thyroid, without a cyst.

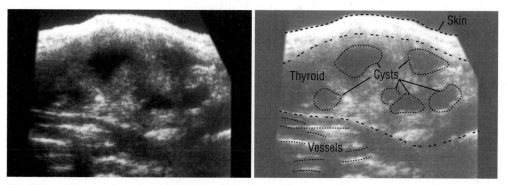

Fig. 252c. Heterogeneous enlarged thyroid with multiple nodules, some of which have undergone cystic degeneration.

Other masses in the neck

Ultrasound is very useful in differentiating masses in the neck and showing their consistency, shape, size, continuity, and relationship with the thyroid and the vascular bundle. The etiology of such masses is not always recognizable.

Abscess

The size and shape of a cervical abscess are very variable, and the outline is often very irregular and unclear. On ultrasound, there are usually internal echoes. In children, abscesses are most commonly in the retropharyngeal region (Fig. 253).

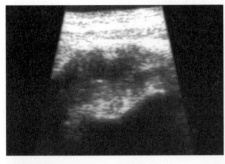
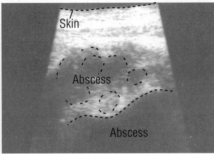

Fig. 253a. Longitudinal scan: a retropharyngeal abscess in a 4-year-old girl.

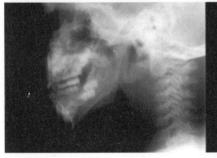
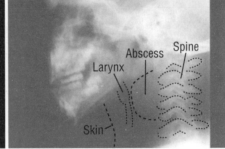

Fig. 253b. A lateral radiograph of the neck, showing the same abscess.

Adenopathy

The diagnosis of enlarged lymph nodes in the neck is usually made clinically, but ultrasound is a satisfactory method of follow-up. On ultrasound, lymph nodes will appear as hypoechogenic masses with regular outlines, solitary or multiple, nodular, oval or round, and variable in size from 1 cm upwards. Ultrasound cannot determine the cause of the lymph node enlargement (Fig. 254).

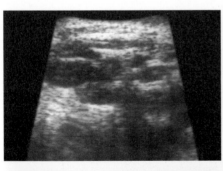
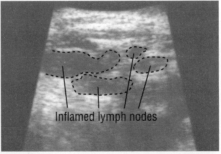

Fig. 254a. Multiple inflamed cervical lymph nodes.

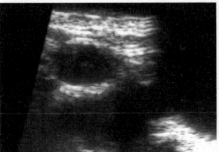
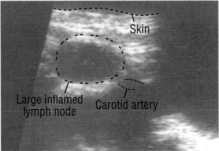

Fig. 254b. Enlarged inflamed lymph nodes near the carotid artery.

Cystic hygromas (lymphangiomas)

These are of variable size, are usually situated laterally in the neck, and may extend to the thorax or axilla. On ultrasound they are fluid-filled, often with septa (Fig. 255).

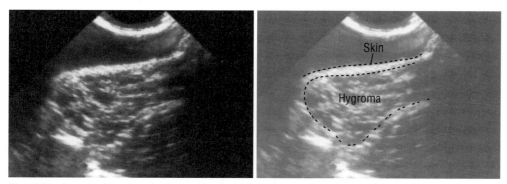

Fig. 255. A cystic hygroma in the neck of a child, with multiple fluid-filled spaces.

Less common neck masses

In children, echogenic masses may be due to haematoma (Fig. 256). In the cervical muscles, a cystic or complex mass may be a thyroglossal cyst (in the midline), a branchial cleft cyst (in the lateral neck) or a dermoid.

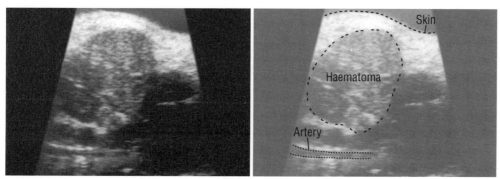

Fig. 256. A haematoma in a child's neck.

Vascular abnormalities

It is possible with ultrasound to demonstrate atheromatous plaques and show stenosis in the carotid artery, but it is not possible to evaluate blood flow without Doppler ultrasound and, in many cases, angiography (Fig. 257).

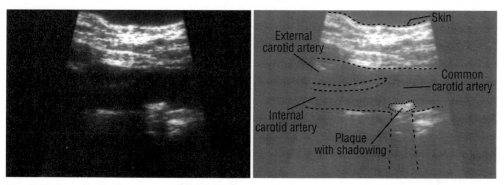

Fig. 257. Longitudinal scan: a calcified atheromatous plaque just proximal to the bifurcation of the left common caroid artery.

Complete occlusion of the carotid or any other artery cannot be demonstrated without Doppler ultrasound.

Notes

CHAPTER 20

Pericardium

Indications

Suspected pericardial effusion. Echocardiography is a very specialized technique. The use of a general purpose ultrasound unit should be limited to the search for a pericardial effusion.

Preparation

1. **Preparation of the patient**. No preparation is required.

2. **Position of the patient**. The patient is examined lying supine (on his/her back) and then in the sitting position.

   Apply coupling agent over the cardiac area.

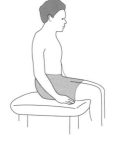

3. **Choice of transducer**. Use a 3.5 MHz transducer. Use a 5 MHz transducer for children or thin adults.

   Use the smallest transducer available to perform intercostal scanning.

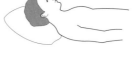

3.5 MHz adults   5 MHz children

4. **Setting the correct gain**. Start by placing the transducer centrally at the top of the abdomen (the xiphoid angle). Angle the beam to the right side of the patient to image the liver. Adjust the gain setting to obtain an image with normal homogeneity and texture. It should be possible to recognize the strongly reflecting lines of the diaphragm next to the posterior part of the liver. The portal and hepatic veins should be visible as tubular structures with an echo-free lumen. The borders of the portal veins will have bright echoes, but the hepatic veins will not.

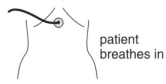

patient breathes in

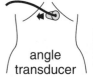

angle transducer   patient holds breath in

Scanning technique

Start with the transducer (with a small acoustic window) centrally in the upper abdomen close to the edge of the ribs (the xiphoid angle).

Angle the transducer towards the head (cephalad) and ask the patient to take a deep breath. This will usually show a transverse section of the heart and the examination can be carried on through the respiratory cycle. If the transducer is small enough to be applied between the ribs, different sections can be obtained. There will usually be masking by the ribs unless the transducer is very small. Blood is echo-free and the cardiac walls are echogenic. The cardiac chambers vary in size depending on the stage of the cardiac cycle (Fig. 258).

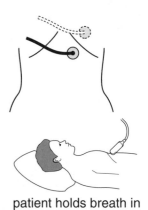

patient holds breath in

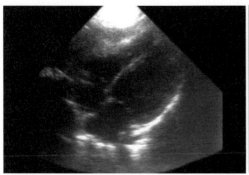
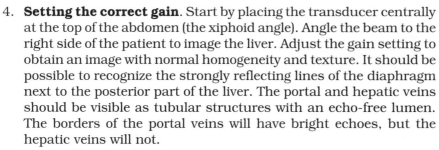
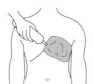

Fig. 258. Transverse scan: the normal heart in diastole.

Pericardial effusion

Fluid around the heart is seen as an echo-free region surrounding the heart muscle (Fig. 259a). (Anechogenic fat anteriorly may resemble fluid.) If there is a small amount of fluid, it can be seen to change in size and position as the heart beats. When there is a moderate amount of fluid, the apex of the heart can be seen moving freely within the pericardial fluid. Cardiac motion may be restricted by a large amount of fluid.

It is not possible to distinguish serous from bloody effusions (Fig. 259b). In malignant and tuberculous pericardial effusions, after the acute stage, there may be localized or loculated effusions caused by adhesions between the two layers of the pericardium (Fig. 259c). Internal echoes in the effusion are due to infection or blood. Suspected calcification within the pericardium is better assessed by radiography.

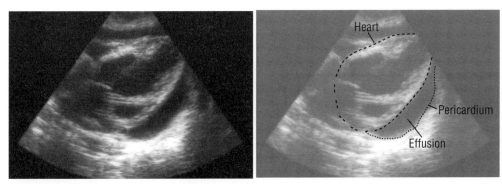

Fig. 259a. A large pericardial effusion.

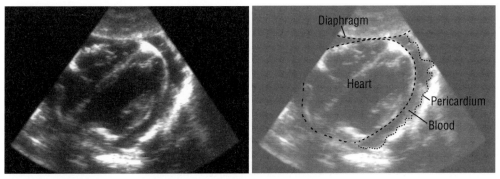

Fig. 259b. Blood in the pericardium (haemopericardium) following trauma.

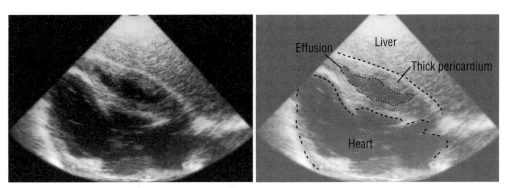

Fig. 259c. A large loculated pericardial effusion.

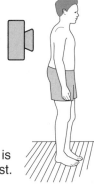

If pericardial calcification is suspected, X-ray the chest.

Notes

CHAPTER 21

Pleura

Indications

Ultrasound can detect pleural fluid and may be helpful in localizing small effusions when aspiration is indicated. If X-rays are already available confirming the pleural fluid, the only reason to use ultrasound is to guide aspiration when the fluid is loculated or there is only a small amount (see pp. 318–319).

> **It is not necessary to use ultrasound to aspirate every effusion.**

Preparation

1. **Preparation of the patient**. No preparation is required.

2. **Position of the patient**. Whenever possible, the patient should be scanned while sitting comfortably.

    Apply coupling agent liberally over the lower part of the chest on the side to be examined.

3. **Choice of transducer**. Use a 3.5 MHz transducer. Use a 5 MHz transducer for children or thin adults. Choose the smallest transducer available in order to scan between the ribs. If only a large transducer is available, there will be shadowing from the ribs, but information can still be obtained.

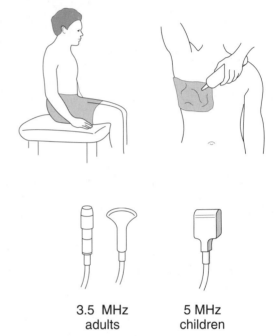

3.5 MHz
adults

5 MHz
children

4. **Setting the correct gain**. Adjust the gain to obtain the best image.

Scanning technique

The transducer should be centred between the ribs and held perpendicular to the skin. Echo-free pleural fluid can be recognized above the diaphragm, lying in the pleural space. The lung will be highly echogenic because of the contained air (Fig. 260).

First scan the suspected area and compare with X-rays if available; then scan at different levels because the effusion may be loculated and is not always in the lower pleural space (the costophrenic angle) (Fig. 260c). Alter the patient's position to see how much the fluid moves.

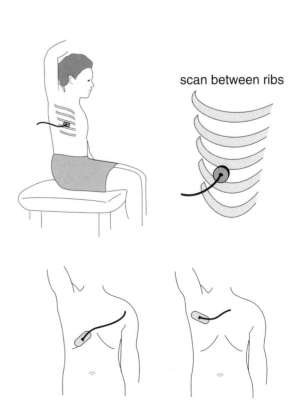

scan between ribs

The abnormal pleura

Pleural effusions are hypoechogenic or slightly echogenic, and sometimes contain thick septa. Liquid blood and pus are also echo-free, but septations may cause reflections (Fig. 260c). It is not always possible to differentiate between fluid and solid pleural or peripheral lung masses (Fig. 260d). Move the patient to a different position and rescan. Fluid will usually move unless there is loculation or an excessive amount. Peripheral lung or pleural masses do not move. Aspiration may be the only way to establish the diagnosis.

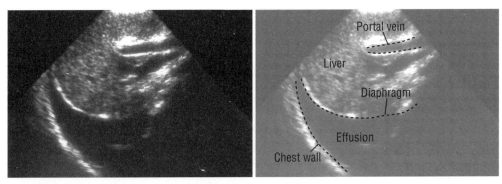

Fig. 260a. Transverse scan: a moderate sized pleural effusion.

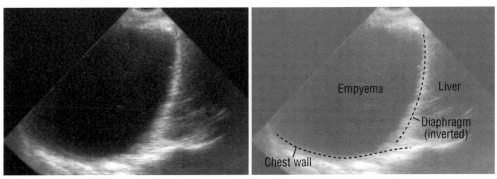

Fig. 260b. Longitudinal scan: a large pleural empyema on the right side.

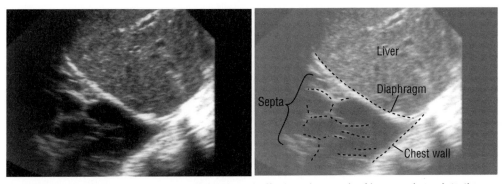

Fig. 260c. A loculated, multiseptate right pleural effusion, the result of haemorrhage into the pleural space.

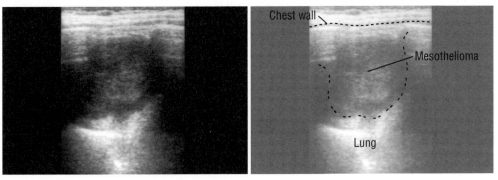

Fig. 260d. A pleural mass (mesothelioma).

Notes

CHAPTER 22

Ultrasound-guided needle puncture

Ultrasound guidance is particularly important for biopsy of a small tumour, or aspiration of a small effusion or abscess which is difficult to localize clinically. It is not necessary to use ultrasound to aspirate every effusion or ascites, but it is important when the fluid or tumour is close to vital organs. Ultrasound should then be used to choose the shortest and safest route for needle insertion.

Ultrasound is an ideal way to guide a needle because the steel reflects ultrasound and can therefore be clearly followed as it enters the body. However, it is possible for only part of a needle to show. This can happen if the front portion of the needle leaves the scanning plane and becomes invisible. The apparent tip is then actually the point at which the needle leaves the scanning plane and is not the *actual* tip of the needle. Not only will this make it impossible to reach the required puncture site, but it may cause damage by puncturing the wrong tissues. Fig. 261 illustrates these difficulties.

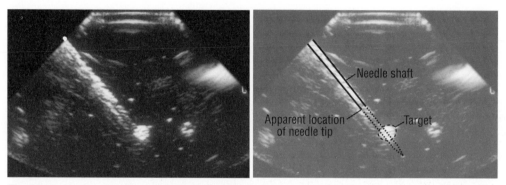

Fig. 261a. An incorrectly angled scan: the point of the needle is not in the scanning plane and is, therefore, not visible. As a result, the needle tip does not seem to have reached the target.

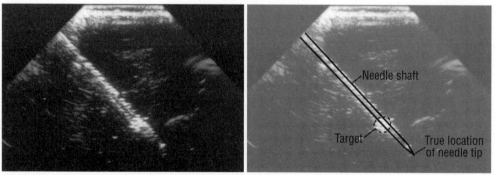

Fig. 261b. A correctly angled scan of the same needle: the needle tip is now in the scanning plane and is clearly visible beyond the target.

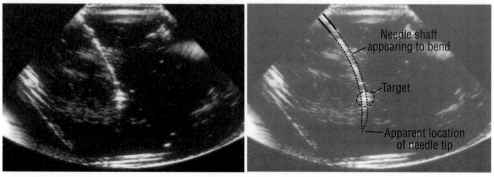

Fig. 261c. Scan of a needle which appears to bend, giving a false impression of the position of the tip.

Images for Fig. 261a–c were obtained using a breast phantom.

Warning: only that section of the needle *within the scanning plane* will appear on the screen. Make sure you can see the *actual* tip of the needle. There may be a significant length that is not imaged.

There are devices to keep the needle in the correct plane of the ultrasound by fastening it to the transducer. When the needle is correctly positioned, the transducer can be disconnected leaving the needle in position.

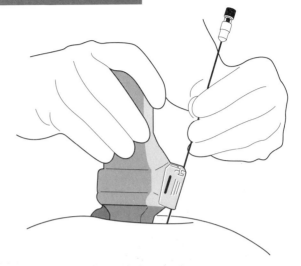

It is always easier to guide a needle into spaces filled with fluid (amniotic fluid, ascites, cysts, abscesses, or pleural effusions) than into solid tissue. The tip of the needle is not always clearly visible in solid tissue: it may be recognized only when moving and be very difficult to see when stationary.

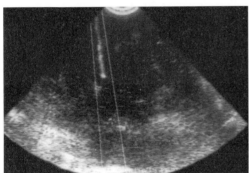 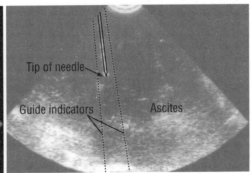

Fig. 262a. Needle aspiration of abdominal ascites, guided by ultrasound.

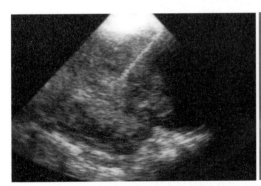 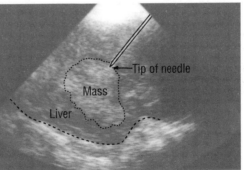

Fig. 262b. Needle biopsy of a mass in the liver, guided by ultrasound.

Whenever possible, fluid should be aspirated from the centre of a cyst, but the necrotic centre of a tumour should be avoided. The most dependent region of pleural fluid should be chosen for aspiration. Once the needle is correctly positioned, ultrasound should be used to monitor the removal of the fluid or cyst contents.

It is very important that guided needle punctures are carried out in strictly sterile conditions.

320

Notes

ANNEX

Specifications for a general purpose ultrasound scanner (GPUS)

Before purchasing an ultrasound scanner, it is essential to decide what types of examination are to be carried out and then exactly what equipment is needed (pp. 18–21). The minimum technical capability expected should be made clear to any potential supplier. A WHO Scientific Group has recommended minimum specifications for a general purpose ultrasound scanner. Some scanners will exceed these specifications but, for general use, any scanner that meets these specifications will produce high-quality scans for all general purpose examinations.

The original GPUS specifications were defined in 1984.[1] The technology of ultrasound scanners has progressed significantly since then, and the original specifications have been reviewed and updated. While there has undoubtedly been progress, not all the new developments are cost-effective or result in better patient care. Any benefits claimed for new technology must be carefully assessed. If necessary, consult an expert ultrasonologist who is aware of your needs.

It is unwise to accept any scanner that does not meet these minimum specifications, even if it is less expensive. Any significant downgrading of the specifications is likely to result in loss of quality.

Specifications

1. The transducer design should be curvilinear (convex) or a combination of linear and sector.

2. The standard transducer should have a central frequency of 3.5 MHz with accurate focusing. An optional transducer of 5 MHz is desirable if it can be afforded. The 3.5 MHz is a fair compromise between penetration and resolution, but the 5 MHz is very helpful in scanning children, thin adults and superficial organs. It is a worthwhile addition but should not replace the 3.5 MHz transducer.

3. The sector angle should be 40° or more, and the linear array should be 5–8 cm long.

4. The controls should be simple and easy to use. Overall sensitivity (gain or transmitter power) and time gain compensation must be an integral part of the circuit. It must be possible to vary the time gain compensation from a preset level. However, this is not essential if the time gain compensation is at the correct level for obstetrics with a preset alternative for the upper abdomen: then more than 80% of patients can be satisfactorily examined by varying the overall gain only.

5. The frame rate must be 15–30 Hz for the linear array and at least 5–10 Hz for the sector array.

6. The frame freeze should have a density of at least $512 \times 512 \times 4$ bits (to provide 16 grey levels).

7. At least one pair of electronic omnidirectional calipers with quantitative readout is required.

8. It must be possible to add patient identification data (hospital number, date of the examination, etc.) to the screen and the final record.

9. It should be possible to obtain a permanent record (hard copy) of the scan. The hard copy unit must work satisfactorily in the same environment as the scanner (pp. 19 and 323).

10. There should be two or three imaging dynamics ranges available for

---

[1] WHO Technical Report Series, No. 723, 1985.

post-processing. It is unnecessary to have a wider range of options.

11. The screen of the video monitor should measure at least 13 cm × 10 cm, preferably larger.

12. The equipment must be portable so that an average adult can move it over at least 100 metres: if on wheels, these must be suitable for rough irregular surfaces, but a unit that can be moved without wheels is preferable.

13. The equipment must be suitable for the local climate, and be protected against dust, damp, extremes of temperature, tropical environments, etc. It should be possible to use the scanner continuously within a temperature range of 10–40 °C and 95% relative humidity.

14. It must be possible to transport or store the unit safely under adverse conditions. It should not be affected by air transport or being moved across rough country in any vehicle. A specially designed case for transport may be necessary.

15. It is essential that the scanner can operate from the local power supply and is compatible with the voltage, frequency and stability of the local current. The equipment should be able to stabilize a voltage variation of ±10%. If there is a greater fluctuation in the local supply (and this should be tested before purchasing the unit), an additional voltage stabilizer should be obtained. These voltage-stability tests *must* be carried out before the scanner is accepted (see p. 21). The equipment should conform to the standards set by the International Electrotechnical Commission for medical electrical equipment, and must be properly earthed (grounded).

16. Many ultrasound scanners incorporate biometric tables in the microprocessor memory. These are useful, but care should be taken to ensure that clinical measurements are made in exactly the same way as was used to provide the tables. Biometric tables may not be universally applicable and should be adjusted for local standards.

17. It is essential to ensure that servicing is available locally. No ultrasound unit should be purchased unless there are trained service engineers available in the vicinity. When in doubt, ask other local users of ultrasound equipment about the quality of the service and maintenance provided. This may well be the deciding factor when choosing between scanners.

> **The most expensive ultrasound unit is one that is not working.**

18. Service manuals and operating and maintenance instructions should be provided at the time of purchase, especially if local servicing is not readily available.

19. Accessories for ultrasound-guided puncture or biopsy must be easy to sterilize.

The above specifications will not be met by the cheapest and simplest scanners. However, any unit that *does* comply with the GPUS specifications will be entirely suitable for all the examinations described in this manual: that is, for 90–95% of the commonest ultrasound examinations. More complicated investigations will require more sophisticated and much more expensive scanners.

Further advice may be obtained from Radiation Medicine, World Health Organization, 1211 Geneva 27, Switzerland.

Notes

Index